More Advance Praise for *Not What the Doctor Ordered*

*"A well-written, interest-grabbing text that tells the reader
all about our health care industry: How it works, what is
wrong with it, how to fix it. Mandatory reading for all
our politicians who, one way or another, are bound and
determined to make the fix. Mandatory reading for
anyone who wants it fixed."*

William K. Coors
Chairman and President
Adolph Coors Company

*"Consumers. Choices. Common sense. These 'three Cs' of
health care have been largely missing from the debate about
health care reform. For a refreshing, easy-to-read and serious
approach to health care reform that does not require new
taxes and large, government bureaucracies, read Jeff Bauer's
provocative* Not What the Doctor Ordered.*"*

Philip M. Burgess
President & Senior Fellow
Center for the New West—Denver, Colorado

*"Jeffrey Bauer is one of today's most creative thinkers in the
health care field; his fresh ideas on the health care system
are now presented in this necessary and timely book."*

Lowell C. Kruse
President
Heartland Health System in St. Joseph, Missouri

Jeffrey C. Bauer

Not What the Doctor Ordered

Reinventing Medical Care in America

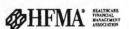 HFMA® HEALTHCARE FINANCIAL MANAGEMENT ASSOCIATION

A 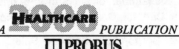 HEALTHCARE 2000 *PUBLICATION*

PROBUS
PUBLISHING

Chicago, Illinois
Cambridge, England

A **HEALTHCARE 2000** *PUBLICATION*

Table of Contents

Foreword

Universal coverage!

Cost containment!

Health insurance security!

Comprehensive benefits!

These may be the cries driving health care reform today, but do they address the underlying causes for what really ails our health care system?

For example, if we are to adopt a new system, will it allow provider choice? Are there enough primary care providers to actually allow universal access even if financial barriers are removed? Will a new health care system address root causes of poor health, such as poverty, environmental hazards, individual behavior patterns, lack of jobs, and lack of hope?

There are no easy answers to these questions, and it's universally assumed that we may need to experiment with multiple panaceas before finding some that truly reform and improve our health care system. Yet in the midst of all this is a simple solution that has been overlooked: the one espoused by Jeff Bauer in *Not What the Doctor Ordered*. Surely, Bauer's remedy is just what the doctor *should* have ordered. It is the only plan I have seen that takes a truly innovative look at improving the system. It clearly allows a choice of providers and by doing so saves billions of dollars. And with those billions imagine what we can do! Address the problems of universal coverage, cost containment, health insurance security, comprehensive benefits—even the root causes of poor health.

Bauer's proposal uses the basic strength that has been instrumental during the past two centuries in helping the United States become a world economic power—the free market. He suggests quite simply that the present physician medical monopoly ought to be dismantled to allow entry into the system by qualified, licensed nonphysician providers.

I have long advocated such an idea, and one analogy I like to draw is this: If you were on the board of directors of a bank, the last thing you would want the president of the bank to do is the teller's job. And yet that is what we are doing in medicine today. We have a system whereby a physician specialist with four years of undergraduate education, four years of graduate education, and three to six years of residency is *legally* the only person qualified to look down a child's throat and prescribe an antibiotic.

One of the beauties of Bauer's plan is that it should please those on opposite ends of the political spectrum. Conservatives will certainly vote for less government intervention and free market competition. Liberals can get excited about how Bauer's system encourages increased patient responsibility, more self-care, and multiple choices for the consumer.

For employers, the plan would mean increased savings that could help U.S. industry compete in the global market. For government payers, the plan would mean new, lower-priced options for all consumers, and enough savings to fund basic coverage for all Americans currently unable to afford care.

If this sounds too good to be true, why are we not even discussing it? The answer lies in the monopoly itself, which has us convinced that the physician alone is capable of delivering health care services. To buttress this belief, my physician colleagues often employ three lines of reasoning:

First, they argue that most people would not want to see a nonphysician provider for health and medical problems. While true in some instances, this claim has often been rebutted, though no less convincingly than by David M. Eisenberg (et al.).[1] Eisenberg pointed out that in 1990, one-half of all Americans sought medical assistance from nonconventional providers, (e.g., massage therapists, energy healers, biofeedback technicians, acupuncturists, hypnotherapists, and other practitioners of not commonly found "cures" in medical schools or hospitals in the United States), for an estimated total of 425 million visits. Eisenberg didn't even factor in some of the presently accepted "conventional" nonphysician providers—dentists, podiatrists, optometrists, and others—who have provided care to millions of people even while competing with the present monopoly.

The second argument some of my colleagues have put forward is that nonphysician providers don't have adequate training to detect serious illness. There is simply no evidence to substantiate this claim. Training for nonphysician providers is already rigorous and is becoming more so every year. Just like doctors, they are taught to recognize problems that fall outside their areas of expertise, as well as when and how to make referrals. Further, they must pass extensive board examinations in order to become licensed and certified. The vast majority of these health care providers are dedicated professionals truly wanting to do what is best for each patient.

The third argument my colleagues use is that opening up the system will not save it money. Refuting this argument is where Jeff Bauer excels. Using pure common sense and easy-to-understand examples, Bauer proves convincingly that a free market system for health care can and will work. *Not What the Doctor Ordered* is an elegant statement on why we simply must take the shackles off America's many competent nonphysician providers.

One simple way of how money can be saved by using nonphysician providers is exemplified in a study done by Dean Ornish, MD.[2] Ornish's use of a lowfat diet, exercise, relaxation, stress management, and group support to control

---

1. Eisenberg, David M., "Unconventional Medicine in the United States" *New England Journal of Medicine*, January 28, 1993: 246-252.
2. "Can Lifestyle Changes Reverse Coronary Heart Disease?" *The Lancet.* July 21, 1990.

cardiac diseases is exactly the type of treatment that trained nonphysicians can administer efficiently. To be able to decrease the amount of open heart surgery even 20% would save billions of dollars and immeasurable suffering. Physicians are trained in the use of medications and surgery, both wonderful modalities for helping people some of the time. But we cannot continue to use them, for both health and financial reasons, to treat every human ailment. Instead, we must allow—even encourage—other healing methods and other providers.

In 1982 in Mankato, Minnesota, a group of health care professionals and I developed the Wellness Center of Minnesota. We had the idea to utilize a diverse group of practitioners—doctors, nurses, physical therapists, counselors, and others—in one setting all working closely together. With stars in our eyes, we moved fearlessly forward knowing the people of the upper Midwest would be incredibly excited about our innovative concept.

In fact, the people were very excited, but third party payers were not. For various reasons, our methodology didn't fit in with their concept of how health care should be administered. Rather than reimburse us for listening to patients' problems and getting to the root of the causes of those problems, and for stressing preventative care, they were more comfortable financing something more tangible—like coronary bypass for a 50-year-old man who smoked and drank too much—even though it was much more expensive.

Despite our nonstandard approach—that is, employing a team of physician and nonphysician providers, all specialists in their own areas, stressing health and wellness rather than waiting to repair illness—our little clinic managed to survive. And out of this concept has emerged a new style of health care clinic we call Lamat, located in the Minneapolis-St. Paul area and based on this same premise.

In this book, Jeff Bauer describes so well how we must push for a new model—a new idea whose time has come. I believe the future holds the exciting possibility that a large number of health care centers similar to what we envisioned with the Wellness Center a dozen years ago and with Lamat today will spring up to provide a new model: A diverse group of practitioners working together as *equals* in a collaborative manner. The goal will be not only be to deliver cost effective and excellent individual care, but also to become centers of community-based care for the promotion of public and preventative health partnerships.

Indeed, Bauer's model gives us a glimpse of how health care will be delivered in the 21st century. No longer will physicians alone define a limited scope of medicine because no longer can practitioners separate the problems they see in their offices from the problems of the community. A new partnership of physicians and nonphysician providers will empower communities to examine and deal with the basic behavioral, social, and environmental problems that are the root of so much disease and infirmity.

Forget the ongoing debate in Congress over who's going to pay for what and how. Instead, read *Not What the Doctor Ordered*. It will soon be the Rx for curing our ailing health care system.

William D. Manahan, M.D.
Mankato, Minnesota

Preface

The new ideas presented in this book are the result of one health economist's uncommonly broad exposure to our medical care delivery system over the past 25 years. A few words about my mostly unplanned career in the health industry will help the reader understand how I came to rethink the very foundations of American medicine. At the same time, I feel a strong sense of obligation to acknowledge several very important people who helped shape my thinking along the way. Of course, none of these individuals can fairly be held accountable for my very different vision of the future of health care in the United States, but they do deserve to be recognized for their influence. They are people who made a difference to me.

Even though I have had many different jobs—including meteorology researcher, professional photographer, consultant, and video producer—my fundamental self-image is that I am a teacher. I was raised for the role. The two most influential role models in my life, my father and his father, were both engineering professors at major universities. The only real career dilemma I ever remember facing was what I would teach—not whether I would teach—as I followed in their footsteps.

The thought of becoming a health economist hadn't even crossed my mind when I began college with the expectation of majoring in physics. Some four years and three majors later, I found myself graduating in May 1969 with a bachelor's degree in economics and a Fulbright Scholarship to study economic development planning in Switzerland. I was also admitted to several graduate schools to study agricultural economics. If the Selective Service had not sent me a draft notice at the same time, I might today be one of the world's leading academic authorities on some arcane subject like the impact of tube wells on wheat production in Asia.

Because I am a pacifist, my draft board sent me to perform two years of alternative service at Penrose Hospital in Colorado Springs, Colorado. My initial assignment was as medical records clerk on the "graveyard" shift, seeming punishment for having just married a nice woman with an 8-to-5 job. The drudgery of that first assignment was quickly curtailed when the hospital's Director of Laboratories recognized me as the freelance photographer whose pictures had appeared occasionally in local newspapers. I had exactly the skills he needed to run the laboratory's division of medical photography, and my salary as approved by the draft board was—much to the pleasure of the hospital's director of finance—less than half the going wage for a professional clinical photographer.

Consequently, I spent the better part of two years working alongside practicing physicians and medical residents who asked me as many questions about photography as I asked them about medicine. I am very grateful to the many wonderful doctors who taught me something about clinical medicine during this period, but I particularly appreciate and acknowledge the extra attention given me by Dr. Morgan Berthrong and the other pathologists at Penrose. In addition to teaching me an incredible amount about the theory and practice of medicine, they also challenged me to consider becoming a physician. They were tempting salesmen, but at that time an assured career in economic development seemed more promising than an uncertain future that would begin with taking the infamous Medical College Admission Test.

My resolve to become an economist prevailed, but the type of economist I was to become was changed unexpectedly and dramatically by Sister Myra James Bradley, Penrose Hospital's CEO and one of the most competent and caring executives I have ever had the pleasure of knowing. She was extremely kind to me from the day I began working at Penrose, occasionally inviting me to the front office for chats about economics in general and health care in particular. I was never sure why she was so interested in economics until the day when she hastily summoned me from the darkroom to attend a meeting with her and Dr. Berthrong. The urgency of the situation arose from the fact that a new piece of laboratory equipment had been installed that morning. The first tests were ready to be run on the machine, but the fee to be charged had not yet been determined.

I silently prepared a mini-lecture on price theory as Sister Myra James explained the problem, but she never gave me the opportunity to express my economist's perspective on the issue at hand. Rather, she reported to Dr. Berthrong that identical machines were now in use in two other hospitals in Colorado: one in Pueblo, 40 miles to the south, where a fee of $10 was being charged, and the other at the medical school's teaching hospital 60 miles to the north in Denver, where the fee was $15. She concluded by proposing a $12 fee at Penrose, justified by the geographic fact that Colorado Springs was somewhere between Pueblo and Denver, but closer to Pueblo. Dr. Berthrong agreed, and the meeting was over. I was somewhat chagrined that I had not been asked to say a word throughout the meeting, but Sister casually said to me as we walked out the door, "See? Health care really needs economists." At that very moment, I felt the calling to become a health economist—whatever that was. I subsequently wrote to the graduate schools that had accepted me in their economic development programs to see if I could specialize in health economics instead.

A private university back east denied my request on the grounds that health economics was not a defined field of study in its economics department. A state university in the Midwest reconfirmed my acceptance because a professor there was interested in the idea of applying economic analysis to the allocation of health care resources, but the admissions office informed me that financial assistance would only be available if I were to remain in the economic development program. (Ironically, I am now a part-time teacher at that university's medical school; I teach doctors how to evaluate clinical literature.) Fortunately, my home state school was willing to give me financial aid independent of my field of study, so I entered the Ph.D. program in economics at the University of Colorado after belatedly completing the Fulbright year in Switzerland at the University of Geneva (where I did the equivalent of a master's thesis on the history of economic development planning in Pakistan— because the Swiss didn't recognize health economics at the time, either).

I am enduringly grateful to four economists who had a profound influence on me at the University of Colorado at Boulder. First, I acknowledge my appreciation for the guided freedom given to me by my academic advisor, Dr. Larry Singell (now Dean of the School of Business). He convinced me of the need to become a good economist first and a health economist second. At his urging, I studied general microeconomic theory with more dedication than I might have otherwise devoted to it. I also served for two years as his teaching assistant, where I absorbed his superb skills in making economics understandable to non-economists. If this book presents at least some economic theory clearly and meaningfully, Professor Singell deserves much of the credit for the accomplishment.

He also directed me toward the late Kenneth Boulding, who became my unofficial mentor (many discussions of his concept of creative tension) and musical collaborator (occasional performances of Medieval and Renaissance recorder music) throughout graduate school. Kenneth did more than any other economist to prepare my mind for the new perspectives embodied in this book. Were it not for Sister Myra James, I would not be a health economist. Were it not for Kenneth Boulding, I would probably be the kind of economist who would find this book to be utterly ridiculous. (More on this subject later.)

Professor Wes Yordon also deserves special mention. He supervised my Ph.D. dissertation on doctors' fee-setting behavior, and he convinced me that I should not treat doctors as a "special case." ("Special case" treatment is the traditional economist's way of justifying government regulation on the grounds that the market forces of economics will not work in a particular market. It is behind most economists' unworkable approaches to health care reform. More on this later, too.) I followed his advice and successfully defended my final thesis before a committee of outside professors, including two from the medical school who were initially concerned that I was studying health care with the same theoretical tools used to explain pricing decisions in competitive industries. This approach was considered somewhat heretical at the time, but as we will see in this book, applying basic economic principles to health care makes sense. We can reform our health care system by promoting competition among qualified independent providers, and we can do it without the increases in taxes and regulation that lurk behind the "special case" solutions being debated in Congress.

The final credit goes to a Harvard economist, Wassily Leontief, who occasionally lectured at the University of Colorado. Following a presentation on his Nobel Prize-winning development of input-output analysis, I asked him to define the role of an economist because I found myself in the awkward position of almost having a Ph.D. in economics but having no concrete idea of what it was that economists were supposed to do once they entered the "real world." Professor Leontief's answer made an indelible impression on my mind. He said a good economist was like a chef who looked in the pantry to identify the available ingredients and then determined all the dishes that could be made from them and the prices that should be charged. I have ever since approached the health economy as a chef, contemplating the different ways that our medical ingredients could be made into different dishes that would satisfy our wants and needs for health care. (In this context, I've always liked the old French saying, "To make an omelet, you must break eggs.") This book effectively represents the resulting menu and explains why my selections from it are different from those that would normally be ordered by a doctor.

Professor Leontief's metaphor is a good illustration of an important concept of conventional economic theory—substitution in consumption. Although a consumer might have a specific purchase in mind, he or she is often willing to accept a close substitute if the qualitative differences in the competing goods are less important than the difference in their prices. For example, many people who would like to buy a Mercury Sable are probably willing to accept a Ford Taurus instead when they determine that the cars are pretty similar in style but significantly different in price. On the other hand, a Taurus is unlikely to be an acceptably close substitute to the well-heeled buyer intending to purchase a Mercedes 450-SEL. This book shows how we can achieve the goals of health care reform—without raising taxes or creating new bureaucracies—by applying the simple economic principle of substitution to the medical marketplace.

I could not have come to recognize the relevance of the substitution effect without the help of doctors. Many of my best friends and relatives are medical doctors, and I truly appreciate the countless hours that they have spent sharing with me their honest assessments of the strengths and weaknesses of American medicine. My plan for reinventing it absolutely must not be construed as a personal vendetta against doctors because most of the doctors I know are totally dedicated professionals—in the proudest sense of that overused term— and thoroughly decent human beings. Doctors will continue to make unique and valuable contributions to our health. They will continue to be the only acceptable choice in those clinical areas where there are no acceptably close substitutes.

However, in my 11 years (1973–84) as full-time teacher and administrator at the University of Colorado Health Sciences Center and in my subsequent career as consulting medical economist and health care futurist,[1] I have also

---

1. Economic training does provide some tools for predicting the future, that is, making statements about what is likely to happen in the future and when it will happen. Economic futurists are known for predicting things like the rate of inflation or the level of unemployment for the coming year. They are also known for being far from 100 percent accurate, which is why Kenneth Boulding once jokingly told me that I should be very careful when making predictions. If I were talking about a specific change that I was sure would happen in the future, he advised me not to give a specific date when the change would occur. On the other hand, if giving the date when a major change was going to happen, I should say very little about what the change would be. "Above all," he told me, "if you forget this advice and tell people both what will happen and when it will happen—and you turn out to be right—don't act surprised."

learned that some nonphysician health professionals are capable of providing many of the caring services that have been the protected domain of medical doctors. Acceptable substitutes for doctors do exist. Therefore, this book is not written as a criticism of doctors, but rather as revelation of a fact they have denied or suppressed: in many aspects of diagnosing and treating illness, doctors are not unique.

A few final credits are in order as I embark on this odyssey. I particularly thank Dr. John Kralewski, my first "boss" when I joined the medical school faculty as a junior member, for giving me multidisciplinary experience in the health sciences. John created the opportunities that got me actively involved in the education of physicians, dentists, nurses, and pharmacists during the years that I was a full-time professor. Dr. Eunice Blair, Dr. Bob Aldrich, Dr. Larry Meskin, Dr. Sholom Pearlman, Dr. John Cobb, and Dr. Peter Dawson were particularly helpful along the way. I also express my appreciation to Chancellor John Cowee, my "boss" during my four years in medical center administration. Dr. Cowee encouraged me to think differently about medical care at times when encouragement was needed most. I also thank David Willis, former editor of *Health and Society: Milbank Memorial Fund Quarterly*. His early suggestions concerning the format of this book have proved invaluable.

Three friends deserve special recognition for their help with research and formulation of some of the examples used to illustrate central themes of this book. Eileen Weis, a nurse with considerable firsthand experience in the delivery of health care, spent many hours tracking down information about the training and qualifications of nonphysician providers. Leigh Pomeroy, old college buddy and fellow writer, provided invaluable assistance in helping me shape and sharpen my arguments in favor of adding competition to the practice of medicine. Kimball Miller, M.D., a practicing internist and pediatrician, was always available to discuss clinical issues and to challenge my thinking as it evolved. All three deserve sincere thanks for their generous assistance along the way, but none of them deserves any blame for this final product. The final words and thoughts are mine alone.

I express my appreciation to the good people at Probus Publishing Company. Kris Rynne deserves extra special thanks for her faith in this project. Without her intervention and guidance, I'd probably still be looking for a publisher. Kevin Thornton merits recognition for superb management of the production process. With its multiple layers, this is the most complicated piece I've ever written, but the entire book fell easily into place under his direction. Finally, Trish Nealon was a helpful editor. I was greatly aided by her suggestions concerning clarification and precision. I would also like to thank Rob Pudim for his artistic contribution; his illustrations help make the point.

Above all, I thank my wife, Chris, and kids—Anna, Frank, and Charlie—for putting up with me while I spent hours and days in seclusion with my thoughts and my Macintosh Powerbook. I used to think that family recognition was somewhat out of place in a preface, but now I know otherwise. They, too, made a lot of contributions and sacrifices for this book. I could not have written it without them.

Jeff Bauer
Hillrose, Colorado

"It's a pretty good zoo,"
Said young Gerald McGrew,
"And the fellow who runs it
Seems proud of it, too."

"But if I ran the zoo,"
Said young Gerald McGrew,
"I'd make a few changes.
That's just what I'd do. . ."

Theodor S. Geisel
(Dr. Seuss)
If I Ran the Zoo

Introduction What This Book Is Not

"I must confess that I regard the invention of pseudo-quantities like the coefficient of correlation as one of the minor intellectual disasters of our time; it has provided legions of students and investigators with opportunities to substitute arithmetic for thought on a grand scale."

Kenneth Boulding

"Most people approach statistics like a blotter. They sop it all up, but they get it all backwards."

Alfred E. Newman (Mad Magazine)

The current battle over health care reform has generated a lot of print (not to mention a lot of talk). Almost all of the discussion is focused on changing the way we pay for medical services and who gets them. As you might surmise from its title, this book presents a very different view of the fundamental changes that must occur in our health care delivery system. Not surprisingly, then, a few comments about what this book is not are appropriate for introducing *Not What the Doctor Ordered*.

1. This book is not full of statistics. A quick review of the voluminous written record of the debate over health reform—the shelves of books, the transcriptions of speeches and television programs, the weekly news magazines, the medical journals, the reports of Congressional testimony, and all the other published sources—reveals a mountain of numbers. Statistics are everywhere. . . 37 million (or is it 41 million?) uninsured Americans, health care at 14 percent of our gross domestic product and going to 20 percent, health expenditures rising at double-digit rates, etc. Indeed, many publications are so full of scary statistics about the problem that the thinking behind the proposed solutions—if there is any thinking—is hard to find.

If statistics alone could show us the way to a better health care system, this book would be unnecessary because no other country in the world has generated so many numbers to describe its health care. The United States is clearly the world's number one producer of health statistics (which may help explain why it is number one in per person expenditures on health care), but it is far down the list in terms of producing healthy people. Somewhere between 15 and 20 modern industrialized ("developed") nations spend less than we do on health care and have much healthier populations—all without relying on statistics to decide how medical services ought to be provided.

Besides getting in the way of thinking, statistics present other dangers. For example, by giving an undue impression of precision, they pave the way for highly complex, data-based schemes to regulate our health economy—along with the creation of large government bureaucracies to collect and report the statistics. The more numbers that are available, the more complicated the solutions seem to get. Perhaps worst of all, statistics are almost never very precise—they just *appear* to be. The health economy is too complex and too dynamic to be measured accurately on a current, "real-time" basis. In fact, most of the key data on our health economy are not ready to be reported until a year or two after they are collected—which means we never have accurate, up-to-date measures of the current situation. Sadly, the people who make our laws act like they believe all the statistics, even though they usually know next to nothing about how the numbers are collected or analyzed.[1] We seem to have forgotten the wisdom of the old saying, "There are lies, damned lies, and statistics."

In writing this book, I decided to follow the advice of two sages who had enormous influence on my own intellectual development—Kenneth Boulding

---

1. If you need introduction to the many abuses of information and statistics within the political process, read William Greider's *Who Will Tell the People* (New York: Simon & Schuster, 1992).

and Alfred E. Newman—to explore some exciting new ideas, not some misleading old statistics. (By the way, my chosen approach is not based on personal fear or loathing of statistics. I like statistics. I still teach the subject to physician graduate students to good reviews, and I am currently writing a book on the statistical analysis of health data. I am simply practicing what I teach: thinking should come first, before the numbers.)

2. This book is not written for health professionals, academicians, and policy wonks.[2] Most of the books and articles about health reform suffer from a common defect. The authors of these publications are health professionals, academicians, and policy wonks who are writing for other health professionals, academicians, and policy wonks. The vocabulary and thought processes of these "insiders" is not readily comprehensible to the general public—the individuals and families who ought to be deciding what they want from their health care system.

If the available writings had served their purpose, we would be well on the way to solving the problem. Obviously, we do not seem to be getting any closer to finding workable solutions. A "sure thing" in the months following President Clinton's inauguration, health reform is now unfocused because the White House has made so many changes in the goals and mechanisms of its health plan, and the polls show that most people are confused about the various proposals. Well, the existing approaches to reform are confusing because the related materials are not written to be understood by normal people. The proposals are complex, untried, and theoretical. And they keep changing. Real people want enduring solutions that make sense, not technicalities. This book tries hard to fulfill that need.

3. This book is not a comparative survey of different national health systems. While much can be learned from the health care systems in other countries, I sincerely doubt that copying some other culture's approach to health care is a productive way to resolve America's health care woes. The chief reason is because other countries are different in ways that dictate dif-

---

2. *Wonk* (syn., policy "junkie") is a new, widely used term for people who make their living as experts providing advice on public policy. In the spirit of the Alfred E. Newman quote at the beginning of this chapter, the reader should note that *wonk* is *know* spelled backwards.

ferent approaches to the delivery and financing of health care.[3] From Canada to Great Britain, Japan to Germany, France to Sweden, each country has its own unique concepts of social welfare, education, and health care.

These other countries have built their national health systems over the past 50 years according to social and political imperatives, not doctors' imperatives. Alone among countries, we Americans have allowed doctors to design our medical care system and oversee its development over the past century. (I must also note that these other countries built their health systems without data-driven health economists.)

Because inquiry into the delivery of medical services in other countries is unlikely to produce much of relevance, this book is based on the premise that the United States needs to find its own solution to the problems of its health care delivery system. Besides, most other countries with "model" health systems are experiencing their own crises in the costs and quality of care. Ironically, the solutions proposed in this uniquely American book may solve some of the problems that are now driving up health costs in other countries. Winston Churchill once declared, "In the long run, you can always count on Americans to do the right thing. . . after they have exhausted all the other pos- sibilities." This book proposes an immediate course of action based on a belief that we Americans together can do the right thing by removing the actual deliv- ery of medical care from the single-handed control of doctors.

4. This book is not an exercise in doctor bashing. In spite of the title and the last sentence of the previous paragraph, this book does not criticize the medical profession. Quite the opposite: it uses modern American medicine as the benchmark for independent practice. In no way do I argue that doctors are bad. (Neither do I argue they are perfect. . . we all have room for improve- ment.) Rather, I argue that some other health professionals are now qualified to see patients on their own—without a doctor's orders—when judged accord- ing to the criteria that doctors have used to protect their control over diagno- sis and treatment. The evolution of medical science and education over the past two or three decades has produced acceptable substitutes that should now

---

3. I strongly recommend Lynn Payer's *Medicine and Culture* (New York: Henry Holt and Company, 1988) as an informative, thoughtful, and entertaining introduction to the ways in which differences in health care delivery systems reflect differences in the cultural perception of health.

be made available in a free market economy. The customer should be free to choose between doctors and nondoctors when they are equivalent. The specific degree of substitution will vary by type of doctor—from none for subspecialists like neurosurgeons to a lot for generalists like family practitioners —but the general concept of substitution must be incorporated into our medical care delivery system. This is *real* health reform.

Now, I do know from lots of firsthand experience that some physicians feel threatened by the ideas contained in this book. Indeed, *Not What the Doctor Ordered* takes direct aim at the economic power doctors have amassed since the turn of the century. Whether their perceived fear is loss of control or loss of a well-funded lifestyle (or both), the result is the same: many doctors will respond defensively to the proposed reinvention of our medical care delivery system because they will not be alone at the top. Such a reaction based on self-interest sadly misses the point. Doctors are not bad, but others have become as good within defined scopes of clinical practice. Revolutionary? Yes. Anti-doctor? Not at all!

Happily, I also know many doctors who support this book's ideas—ideas that are long overdue in coming to the forefront of the debate over health care reform. Many physicians have worked hard in recent years to help their qualified nonphysician peers. They have often done so quietly for fear of raising the wrath of other doctors, but they have done so sincerely and deserve to be recognized for their role in helping the legitimate competition. Many physicians already see the opportunity in creating high-quality choices for the American public. I have no doubt that these doctors, although they will no longer be "the only game in town," will be leaders in the development of new and exciting innovations in the way we Americans receive our health care.

These four things, then, are what this book is *not*. Let's see what it *is* by taking a fresh look at the problem with medical care in the United States.

Chapter One

The Monopoly

Monopoly *A market structure with only one seller of a commodity. In pure monopoly, the single seller exercises absolute control over the market price at which he sells, since there is no competitive supply of goods on the market. He can choose the most profitable price and does so by raising his price and restricting his output below that which would be achieved under competition. Monopoly thus leads to a higher selling price, a lower output, and excess profits. Usually, the term monopoly is extended to include any firm or group of firms which act together to fix prices or output.*[1]

This is a book about monopoly, pure and simple. It is a book about a monopoly that exerts great influence over our everyday lives. One that we take for granted. One that we have been conditioned to trust, without question. One that we proudly proclaim as the best in the world. Yet one that uses its power to deprive us of alternatives we would demand if only we knew more about them.

This is a book about a monopoly that controls our very well-being, ushers us into life, and excuses us into death. A monopoly whose highly skilled, dedicated workers do with us as they please because they know our alternative is having nothing done at all. The monopolists repair us and stitch us together,

---

1. *McGraw-Hill Dictionary of Modern Economics* (New York: McGraw-Hill, 1965), p. 331.

have us swallow endless quantities of brightly colored pills, make us endure boring sojourns in sterile cubicles where room service gives us what the monopolists—not the customers—want. They put us at the mercy of expensive machines while saying, "Trust me."

And these monopolists expect us to trust them, without complaint, because they have extensive training and experience and believe no one else can do the job. It's as if all the mechanics work for the same repair shop—the only one around. We are at their mercy because we can't speak their language when it comes to doing the body work.

The practitioners of this monopoly demand great respect *and* relative wealth. We have given them special titles, and we have built for them—at their request and to their specifications—great temples in which to perform their rituals. In fact, we have given them virtually everything they ever wanted and pooled vast public and private resources in order to keep them happy.

Their monopoly is so beloved and so respected that we encourage our children to join its ranks. To have one of *them* in our family is a great honor, indeed. And why not? Acceptance into the monopoly is a ticket to guaranteed employment and a good income. To country clubs, second homes, yachts, ski vacations, tax write-offs, investment portfolios, real estate deals, private schools for their children, etc.

We, the customers, are addicted to the monopoly. We think we need it for our very survival, so we are not inclined to question its established order. We know no other dealer who can meet our needs. And for this addiction, like many addictions, we pay dearly.

This monopoly has a long and proud heritage. It is steeped in an historical tradition of altruism. Not so very long ago, it provided its service for whatever the customer could afford to pay. As will be shown in later chapters, the monopolists even resisted when our government imposed a payment mechanism that set aside money in advance—as much money as the monopolists said they would need. We grew to accept this monopoly and the need to pay for it without a second thought, even institutionalizing mechanisms to keep the cash flowing.

Few of us realize the monopoly is a twentieth century invention. Before it secured monopoly status, its members were only one among many different types of body mechanics. The monopolists did clearly offer the best alternative among those choices available in the early decades of this century. But much has changed since then. Knowledge and technology are propelling our society at warp speed into the twenty-first century. Because of these changes and the opportunities they have created, we now have a demand for adding years to our lives. The monopolists have responded, admirably and profitably.

New choices have arisen in the final decades of the twentieth century—choices just as valid as the one on which the monopoly was founded in the early 1900s. These new choices share the monopoly's proud tradition of human caring and curing, but they are not locked into the monopoly's economic ways of high prices and excess profits. Best of all, the potential competitors are already in existence, already well established, already performing many of the same services as the monopolists. Indeed, the monopolists themselves use many of their potential competitors' services.

But because of the monopoly and of our unquestioning faith in it, these alternatives are rarely available for direct sale to the general public. In almost all cases, only the monopolist can go to the wholesale warehouse to buy and repackage products made by the competition. Competitors are allowed to exist and to perform their services, but only under orders and with permission of the card-carrying members of the monopoly.

The monopoly, of course, is the medical establishment: doctors, physicians, MDs and DOs—the men and women (mostly men) we must see in order to receive all but the most basic medical attention. Only in a very few instances are nondoctors outside the monopoly allowed to diagnose and treat patients on their own without a doctor's order. This situation was justifiable at the beginning of the twentieth century. It is indefensible at the century's end.

What's Wrong with Monopoly?

The rise and fall of monopolies is part of the American way of life, a central theme throughout our economic history. Indeed, the United States was created as a reaction to the British monopoly over Colonial American trade. Under cries of "freedom" and "liberty," American revolutionaries launched their struggle against British control to establish not only a nation where "all men are created equal," but also a nation whose citizens were free to buy what they wanted from whomever they wished. If our ancestors had been more receptive to the monopoly imposed by King George III, we just might be getting our medical care under the British National Health Service. A quick review of the harms of monopoly will help us understand why we should be concerned about the uniquely American medical monopoly that we got instead.

New ideas, new technologies, and new industries almost immediately generated tremendous economic growth in the "new world." Ironically, monopolies arose just as quickly as a natural outgrowth of unregulated capitalism in our new nation's *laissez-faire* economy. Given the role of government in our lives today, we forget too easily that federal intervention in the economic affairs of our country was expressly rejected by the founding fathers. Our future was left to the control of the "invisible hand" of the marketplace, so wondrously described in the year of our nation's independence by Adam Smith in *The Wealth of Nations*.[2] Government regulation was intentionally rejected by the Constitutional Convention. *Caveat emptor* (buyer beware) and the laws of supply and demand were the prevailing rules of commerce for a new nation excited about its future.

Well, we needed almost exactly one hundred years to learn that completely unregulated markets do not produce the happy economic outcomes promised by Adam Smith and other free-market economists. Leaving the economy totally under the direction of the "invisible hand" allowed—you guessed it—the creation of monopolies. Monopolies took control in iron and steel, railroads, agriculture, oil and gas, and other sectors of the nineteenth century American economy. After driving out the competition with various strong-arm business

2. Adam Smith, *An Inquiry into the Nature and Causes of the Wealth of Nations*, originally published in 1776; now available in the Modern Library Edition (New York: Random House, Inc., 1965).

practices, the monopolists took total control. They could get away with charging high prices because consumers had no choice. Either buy from the monopolist at high prices well above actual costs of production, or get along without!

Our nineteenth century experience taught us the ironic lesson that unregulated competition ultimately killed competition, the exact opposite of the outcome that Adam Smith said would be produced by the "invisible hand." We learned that some regulation is necessary to protect competition. (My favorite analogy is to think of the regulator as the referee in sports. Players cannot be expected to play fairly on their own; someone with authority has to make sure that the game proceeds according to the rules.) Recognition of this problem caused Congress to pass the first federal law against monopolies, the Sherman Antitrust Act of 1890. To this day, the Sherman Act is used to fight against restraints of trade that might lead to monopoly outcomes—uncompetitive pricing and restricted choice. The law has serious teeth. Convicted violators can be sent to jail and required to pay fines equal to three times the actual damages caused by the illegal monopoly behavior.

The Clayton Act was passed in 1914 to strengthen the fight against powerful trusts, complementing the Sherman Act's ability to break up existing monopolies by giving the federal government additional tools for preventing the accumulation of harmful market power. The Clayton Act outlawed practices that might allow a business to become a monopoly—practices like price discrimination, interlocking directorates, and tied buying requirements.[3] The Federal Trade Commission was also created in 1914 to serve as a marketplace referee with the power to put an end to "false, fraudulent, misleading, and deceptive" trade practices. Other laws have been passed since then in an effort to keep the free exchange of goods and services just that—free. And to keep markets truly competitive.

---

3. Price discrimination is the practice of charging different prices to different customers for the same good, i.e., charging each customer as much as he or she is willing and able to pay. Interlocking directorates give competing companies a "behind closed doors" opportunity to agree on pricing products and dividing markets—outcomes that should be determined in the marketplace, not the boardroom. Tied buying arrangements require consumers to purchase goods they do not want in order to buy the goods they need; the needed good may be priced reasonably, but the buyer pays extra by being forced to spend money on the unwanted (and usually overpriced) good. All these practices result in consumers paying more and/or buying less than they would in truly competitive markets.

Before we look specifically at the medical monopoly, we need to consider the exception that proves the rule. Monopolies are allowed to exist in some industries with very high fixed-investment costs because competition would lead to higher prices. Natural gas suppliers, electric power generators, and telecommunications companies are monopolies, but with a difference. Their pricing and investment decisions must be approved by a body representing the public interest, called a public utilities commission in most states. These "natural" monopolies are allowed to exist, but they are not allowed to charge whatever they want and to expand or contract at will. Their business decisions must get the approval of appointed or elected officials who serve the public interest.

By far, the largest regulated monopoly in the recent past was the American Telephone and Telegraph Company. Until the mid-1980s, AT&T and its regional subsidiaries were virtually synonymous with our nation's telephone system. Some small companies were allowed to provide phone service in remote areas considered uneconomic by the telephone giant, but "Ma Bell" had no competition in urban or long-distance markets.

Why was AT&T allowed to be a monopoly for so long? Because simple economic analysis indicated that telephone costs would be higher if competitors were allowed to enter the market. Other companies installing their own telephone lines would add enormous costs, which would be passed on to customers through higher phone bills. As long as telephone calls had to be carried over very expensive networks of poles and wires, one large telephone company made a lot more economic sense than several smaller ones. And we were willing to accept this monopoly as long as public utilities commissions had the rate-setting power to prevent AT&T from making monopoly profits at the expense of consumers.

Well, technological progress put an end to the economic reason for the telephone monopoly. Satellites and computers began to replace telephone lines and mechanical switches, dramatically lowering the costs of telecommunications. Our telephone calls began to travel through the air—not over wires. Once the mode of transmission moved from expensive wires to free air, having one telephone company made about as much sense as having one television network. Ma Bell no longer had a good argument for keeping competitors out of the telephone business. In 1982, AT&T consented to its own dismantling, and the rest is history.

No one knew for sure what changes would be in store for the future of telecommunications when AT&T lost its monopoly power. Some commentators predicted that allowing competitors into the market would lead to dire consequences like bad service and higher prices, yet a decade later the result is almost as if the monopoly had never existed. MCI, Sprint, and a host of other long-distance carriers use lower prices to compete with AT&T for our long-distance dollars. (Indeed, MCI and Sprint have captured one-third of the market in just 10 years.) Dozens of regional and local phone companies provide what is acknowledged as the best telecommunications network in the world. Cellular communications companies offer another alternative, giving us instant access to almost anywhere in the world no matter where we are. Meanwhile, the Baby Bells often go head-to-head in the same markets with their former Momma Bell—not only in telecommunications, but in consumer goods and entertainment as well.

The beneficial result of ending AT&T's monopoly is obvious. Absolutely no one is talking about going back to a single telephone company. Today, like never before, we can choose from a dizzying array of communications choices, many unavailable—or even unthinkable—just a few years ago. Actually, AT&T's Bell Labs had already developed many of the new products that have been brought to market since the breakup of Ma Bell, but most of them were not commercialized in the absence of competition. Public utilities commissions could veto big rate increases, but they could not force AT&T to bring new products to market. Faxing is now a way of life, along with portable cellular phones and modems that link our computers via the information highway. We now can buy a $10 telephone and plug it in ourselves without fear of going to jail.[4]

---

4. A note for readers under 30 years of age: ridiculous restrictions were placed on telephone users before the breakup of the telephone monopoly. Until 10 years ago, we had to lease our telephones and pay a high fee to have the wires connected to the little box on the wall. The Bell System did provide good service, but not cheaply, and not always with a friendly smile.

Would the new technologies and services have reached the market as quickly and as inexpensively if our telecommunications system was still controlled by a monopoly? No. Monopolies lead not only to high prices. They also deprive consumers of choice and restrain the introduction of new technology. Monopolies are anticompetitive, pure and simple.

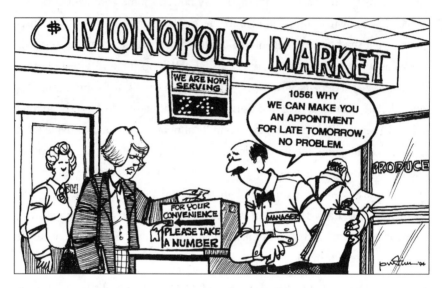

If you are unconvinced by the example of the telephone monopoly, look at the U.S. Postal Service. Where it once held a virtual stranglehold on all parcel delivery, it has in the last two decades yielded considerable market share to aggressively competitive companies like UPS, Federal Express, Emery, and DHL. In the package business, at least, the U.S. Postal Service has been forced to be competitive. Again, the result of competition has been better service and more choices, coupled with prices set by the give-and-take of the free market. The federal government had maintained for decades that the cost of sending a package would rise and the quality of service would fall if competitors were allowed to enter the market. We now know better. *We ought to be suspicious of monopolies that continue to justify their existence by resorting to the argument that price will rise and quality will fall if some other provider of the same service is allowed to enter the market.* Nobody, not even doctors, ought to be exempt from an occasional challenge to the arguments used to keep competitors out of the market.

Do Doctors Really Have a Monopoly?

We may have difficulty thinking of our family doctor as a monopolist. He hardly seems like the nasty robber baron that led to the need for our nation's antitrust laws.[5] He is concerned about our pain and suffering, efficient with his diagnosis, confident in his remedy. The doctor is someone we would like to have as a friend and neighbor. In this sense, the doctor is very much like any other professional—yet this is where the similarity stops, because his profession enjoys a unique status unlike that of an accountant, architect, lawyer, insurance agent, or realtor. Let's examine the differences.

One big difference that sets the American doctor apart from other professionals—and from his pre-World War II predecessor—is that today's typical consumer pays little or none of the doctor's bill. Considerably more than half of all doctors' bills are paid by third-party insurers. Many Americans not only never know, but never have to pay, the full cost of seeing the doctor. They may have to pay deductibles and co-payments, but few ever pay the full cost of service out-of-pocket.

Responsibility for payment predominately rests in the hands of a *third party:* an insurance company, the government, or an employer. Because of this arrangement, price is rarely a determining factor in the patient's personal choice of physician. More often than not, the patient doesn't even know the price of medical services until after the third party has been billed.

Receiving the service first and learning the price later is unique to the medical profession. It brings to mind the days when the practice of medicine was inseparable from the practice of religion. Saving one's soul and saving one's body were both services of the resident priest or priestess until a relatively late date in human history. Religious leaders never charged a set fee to all comers; reimbursement was voluntary and based on ability to pay. Up until the advent of private health insurance only 50 years ago, doctors—like clerics—based

---

5. I apologize for being sexist here, but *he* is the appropriate pronoun to use for this part of my analysis. The medical monopoly is a product of the "good old *boys*," literally. Doctors effectively eliminated women from the medical profession at the same time they eliminated competitors to the medical profession. This chapter in the history of American medicine is regrettable; the profession (and, by extension, the American public) has suffered from the lack of a female perspective. However, the profession can be proud of its recent successes in bringing women back into medicine. Approximately half the students in medical schools now are women.

their fees on whatever the patient could afford. If the patient was wealthy and could pay the doctor's full fee, the full fee was charged and full payment was expected. If all the patient could offer was a dozen eggs or a cord of wood, that became the fee. While the doctor charged whatever the market would bear, the patient paid what he could afford—and both parties were satisfied.

But this all changed with the institutionalization and proliferation of health insurance, both private (e.g., Blue Cross Blue Shield, Aetna, Prudential, etc.) and public (e.g., Medicare and Medicaid), in the years following World War II. Suddenly, the doctor no longer needed to consider the patients' ability to pay. He could charge everyone the same fee—which had been set high enough to compensate for patients who could not pay—*and get reimbursed by the insurance companies or the government for all of it.* (A rare case of having one's cake and eating it too!) In the process, the doctor lifted his income and social standing from middle class to solidly upper crust. Such gains are consistent with the exercise of monopoly power.

While it would make a wonderful "B" movie script to accuse the doctor of manipulating all this for his own benefit, it would not be fair or accurate. In fact, American physicians were brought into this third-party payer system kicking and screaming. Through the American Medical Association (AMA), the physicians' trade organization, doctors consistently opposed any third-party intervention between themselves and their patients on the grounds that money should not influence a doctor's decision on the best treatment for his patient.

Private insurance evolved from its American beginning in the 1930s as organized medicine's compromise with strong political forces pushing for socialized medicine. (Actually, health insurance was invented a half-century earlier in Germany. The idea of health insurance was very slow to catch on in this country precisely because it came from Germany—our mortal enemy in World War I.) Doctors fought strenuously against health insurance for the first three decades of this century. Private health insurance did not really become acceptable until World War II when wage controls prevented employers from giving raises but allowed nontaxable fringe benefits, including health insurance.

When Medicare and Medicaid were proposed during the mid-1960s to cover people who did not get insurance by virtue of employment, organized medicine was the most vocal and powerful opponent. Doctors did not want any government intrusion into the sacred doctor-patient relationship.

Indeed, doctors were so strongly opposed to health insurance that they only accepted it when they discovered that they could control the health insurance industry by controlling the insurance companies. In virtually every other country of the world at this time, including Germany, the health insurance industry was either wholly owned or totally regulated by government. In the United States, it was controlled by doctors. During the 1930s, the Blue Shield system was created of doctors, by doctors, and for doctors as a defensive move to make sure that health insurance followed doctors' orders. In other words, doctors were only willing to accept health insurance if they controlled it. (Does this sound like monopoly behavior? You do not need to have a Ph.D. in economics to answer this question correctly, although you should credit organized medicine for tempering its economic self-interest with a sincere belief that a patient's ability to pay should not influence the doctor's diagnosis or treatment.) Also, patients were more likely to accept monopoly if they didn't have to pay for it because insurance picked up the tab. Isn't this nice little arrangement an appropriate issue for health care reform?

The American doctor may have been forced against his will into the third-party payer system, but ultimately accepting it assured monopoly fees for his services, institutionalized his noncompetitive pricing structure, and gave him a nice standard of living. Organized medicine initially tried hard to kill the goose that would lay golden eggs for its members; now, doctors are struggling just as hard to protect it.[6] They may have become monopolists by accident, but they have become monopolists nevertheless, and they do not want to lose what economic power they have. Doctors have gained the ultimate in monopoly, a seller's market, and they don't want any other sellers of substitute services to have the right to enter the market and sell for less.

---

6. As I write this paragraph on May 5, 1994, *The Wall Street Journal* announces in an article on page B7 that the AMA just introduced a plan to preserve fee-for-service medicine, the hallmark of the Blue Shield payment system. Although the context of the AMA's position has changed, the central argument is what one would expect of a monopolist: we'll begrudgingly allow members of the fraternity to compete on price, as long as no outsiders are allowed to enter the market.

Consumers are understandably bothered by doctors' monopoly power when they stop to think about it, but they are not used to thinking about competitive remedies to the problem. Sadly, the current debate over health reform has focused almost exclusively on government regulation, forcing people to choose among alternative approaches to overseeing the monopoly. This book presents the superior alternative of nurturing fair competition—something quite different from the tired theme of trying to solve our health care crisis by regulating the monopoly.

The evolution of the third-party payer system has distanced the doctor and the patient from true market forces in an otherwise free-market system. This is the way our medical system operates, and so we have become used to it. Unless we are very old or very creative, it's hard for us to remember or imagine a *different* system. But now that other health professionals are qualified and available to compete with doctors, we need to understand how far the medical marketplace has strayed from the proud ideals of our free-market economy. And we need to understand how a different system can be created. We will do both in the following pages.

Ironically, the debate over health reform is indirectly drawing our attention to the failings of the solutions proposed by politicians because the major plans would have the consumer pay more of the health care bill; the 20 percent patient co-payment requirement in the Clinton Plan is typical. We as individuals will be all the more interested in doing something about the high prices of health care if Congress should pass health reform with a mandatory 20 percent patient co-payment, but what can we do? We have become used to the system. Health insurance has insulated us from the problem of the medical monopoly. Lacking a vision of a competitive solution because we have no experience with competition in health care, *we spend endless hours discussing payment reform, looking for new ways to pay the doctor rather than looking for someone else who can sell us the same product or an acceptable substitute for less money.*

The way we are approaching health reform is misdirected and unproductive because it does nothing to break up physicians' monopoly on medical practice. If successful, health reform as proposed thus far (mid-1994) will lead to nothing more than a different way to pay doctors. Even if we are successful in finding new ways to pay them, doctors will still be monopolists if we do not also create a competitive market for health services. The real solution is to open up the market to other health professionals who are qualified to do much of what doctors do.

Just as we realized 10 years ago that a single telephone company was no longer the best way to provide communications, we must now understand that doctors are no longer the only people who can diagnose and treat many of our ailments. Nonphysician providers already treat patients, but they are under doctors' control. The time has come to remove that control and give patients direct access to these qualified providers—nurse practitioners, nurse midwives, physical therapists, pharmacists, and others identified in the following pages of this book. It's time to give doctors some competition by freeing subordinates who have developed the skills to stand on their own and who can provide a quality product at a competitive price. We, the patients, deserve the right to buy direct—to be free to choose between doctors and equally qualified nonphysician health professionals.

So far, the battle over health reform has been fought on the wrong issue. Our policy makers have been seduced into a debate over new and different ways to finance the health care system controlled by doctors. Indeed, the AMA's loud protestations against health care reform remind me of ol' Brer Rabbit begging not to be thrown into the briar patch. Payment reform is a red herring, mystery fans. We really ought to be talking about consumer choice instead, but we cannot expect doctors to raise the subject. The ruling king never likes a challenge to the old order.

Chapter Two

Food
for Thought

Surely, we will end up where we are headed if we do not change direction.

Confucius

Let's say you have just moved to a new town. In the midst of your unpacking you suddenly have this great craving for bananas. So you drive to the nearest supermarket. Even before you walk in, you realize this is a different type of store. It looks nice, but expensive. You hesitate, but you're really intent on getting those bananas, so you check your wallet to make sure you have a few dollars (you do) and walk in.

Immediately a clerk greets you at the door. "What section would you like?" she asks.

"Uh, produce," you say. "I'd just like a bunch of bananas."

"Right this way," she smiles, and heads off down an aisle. You follow, making a mental note that the store has quite a selection. Must be incredibly expensive.

Soon you find yourself in the produce section. "I think I can find them now," you say as you thank the clerk.

"That's all right," she says. "Manager Thompson will be with you in a second. He'll select them for you."

"Manager Thompson?" you think to yourself. "Uh, Miss," you begin, but she's quickly off to assist another customer. It only takes you a second to find those bananas, and boy, are they beautiful. But there's no price on them. Well, okay. You have this craving for bananas and you reason, "How much could bananas cost anyway?" So you pick up a bunch and set off in search for a cashier.

You hardly get two steps before a pleasant voice asks, "Might I help you?" You know right away from the name tag that this is Manager Thompson.

"Just getting some bananas," you say.

"Oh," he says, looking puzzled. "Well, usually I select the bananas for the customer, but it looks like you did pretty well, so I'll just tag these for you."

"Oh," you say, glancing at the tag as he affixes it to your bananas. It bears a long series of numbers. "By the way," you continue, "how much are these?"

"I'm not sure," he says, "you'll have to ask one of the clerks. Excuse me, I have another client."

You reason that bananas can't cost that much, so you head for the checkout stand. The cashier rings it through. "We'll just bill your insurance company," she says.

"Insurance company?" you ask.

"You do have food insurance, don't you? Or are you on the government plan?"

"Government plan?" you ask.

"Uh, perhaps you would rather we just bill you."

"Bill me? For a bunch of bananas?"

"Cash? Well, we do take cash. We realize a few people like to pay that way. We even give a discount." She smiles.

"Cash. Yes, I'll pay cash," you say, beginning to wonder if you're not on a different planet. "Uh, how much is it, anyway?"

"Seven dollars and twenty cents, with the discount."

"*Seven twenty?*"

"We do take credit cards now, if that's easier."

"Uh, yes," you stammer. "Let's do the credit card."

Half an hour later you're back at your new home, dead tired. You treat your-self to a couple of bananas and fall into bed, resolving that you probably won't step foot in that store again.

The next morning you wake up and decide to do some real shopping. But after driving around your new town all morning, you cannot find a store that is not part of the same system. Sales clerks direct you to the various store departments, all of which have at least one manager. Those managers select all your items. The prices aren't readily available; when you do find them, they're exorbitantly high. And the cashiers ask you about food insurance or some government plan, or offer to bill you in a month.

Suddenly, you panic. If bananas are selling for $8 a bunch ($7.20 with the dis-count), you're never sure what anything else might cost until you get the bill, or at least arrive at the checkout stand. Needless to say, you shop very, very sparingly and resolve to write your congressional representatives immediately.

Meanwhile, pausing in one of the stores to remove a few items from your shop-ping list, you notice a woman having her cart filled by one manager after another, seemingly oblivious to the cost of any of the items being selected for her. You follow her around the store and watch in awe as caviar, filet mignon, expensive cheeses, and so forth pile up in her cart. Finally, you can't help yourself. "Excuse me," you say, "but I couldn't help noticing that price seems to be no object for you. I don't want to be forward, but how can you possibly afford it?"

She looks at you strangely and says, "Why, I have food insurance, don't you? My husband and I don't even see the bill. It goes straight to the insurance company. My husband gets it through his work. It's part of his benefits. And you know what's best about it?" She leans forward and looks you in the eye. "It's tax-free! It's like having extra income without having to pay taxes on it! Bye. Nice chatting with you." And she moves on to the candy aisle, where a box of triple cream chocolate-covered cherries is dropped into her cart by yet another friendly manager.

You don't need long to figure out how the system works, and within a few weeks you find a job with a company that offers food insurance. Suddenly you think nothing of buying that bunch of bananas...or anything else. You find yourself fitting right into your new town, having joined the majority of grocery shoppers who, like you, are steering carts full to overflowing. Gone are the days when you agonized over the cost of lettuce, debated whether you could afford a cheap frozen pizza, paused before buying a bunch of bananas. A friendly manager simply places into your cart whatever you need.

And the service is spectacular. Each small section of the store has its own manager. "Hi, I'm Manager Steiner. I'm head of the citrus fruit section." "Hi, I'm Manager Dooley. I take care of the lobsters." "Hi, I'm Manager Kelley. I've got some great gourmet frozen dinners for you." They are all happy, smiling, eager to help you fill your cart—and thoroughly skilled at doing so. "I'm hungry," you say. And they say, "Well, looks like you need some of these hot-house grown tomatoes." Or: "Say, it appears that this free-range chicken will do just the trick."

You learn quickly that their recommendations depend on what section of the store you're in. In the bakery section it's baked goods; in the vegetable section, vegetables; and so forth. Wander into the wrong department with the simple question, "Gee, I'd really like some bananas; could you tell me where they are?", and you're likely to get the response, "No, I'm sorry, bananas aren't what you need; you really should have some of these imported chocolates." And plop! Into your cart they go.

You think back to the old days in your old town. What a big difference this is from a Safeway, Kroger's, or A&P. "The service here is really great," you tell the dairy manager one day as he stuffs your cart with fancy French cheeses. "It has to be," he smiles, piling in some gourmet ice cream for good measure.

"That's how we make our living. We get paid depending on how much we can put in your cart. It's kind of like working on commission, but we call it 'fee-for-service' food." Suddenly it dawns on you: *Commissioned sales without consumer resistance!* What a brilliant idea! And all guaranteed by an insurance company or the government.

"What a beautiful system!" you blurt out.

"Oh, yes," the manager says, "we think it works well. The best in the world, in fact."

"As long as you have insurance," you say, almost without thinking.

The manager smiles and nods, and turns to help another customer. But as you begin to walk away another question comes to mind, and you can't help asking it. "What if I don't have insurance or the government plan? What then?"

The manager shrugs. "It isn't our problem."

You decide to go elsewhere. You want to choose your own food. "Could you please direct me to a store where I can shop for myself?"

"Sorry." He replies. "Not possible. Our chain is the only one licensed to sell groceries."

&. &. &.

I concocted this little scenario to open our minds to new thoughts about the medical market (literally and figuratively), much like a good appetizer opens our taste buds to the flavors of the main course to follow. We would all be astounded if we encountered this situation when we went out to buy groceries. We would rebel at discovering we had no real choice when it came to purchasing something as basic as food—even if we did not have to foot the bill—because we have grown to appreciate both the opportunity to choose among competing grocery stores and the ability to make our own selections off the shelf.

The time is right for us to demand competitive options for purchasing our medical care. Willing and qualified competitors are now available to sell us acceptable, competitively priced substitutes for many of the products that have only been available at the doctors' store. In addition, consumers are ready for the freedom to choose. The pieces of a reinvented health care system already exist. Sadly, we do not know how they could be put together because we have never known any system other than the one described metaphorically in this chapter. The next chapter explains how we got to where we are now, laying foundations for the vision and the plan to move us in a different and better direction for the future.

Chapter Three

Disordered Beginnings: Roots of the Medical Monopoly

The fascinating feature of primitive medicine is that it represents a medical system utterly different from our own, yet one that functions satisfactorily.

Erwin H. Ackernecht, M.D.

Too often we tend to think that if something—be it a landscape, a building, a city, a person—is a certain way, it has always been that way. Meeting someone in his or her later years of life is a prime example. Unless something about the person's past is revealed to us, we tend to think of the new acquaintance only as she or he is today. In many cases, we could be in for a real surprise if we delved into the person's past. It might be something very different from the impression we get based on how the person looks today.

The history of medical care delivery is a good example of something very different from what we might expect based on current appearances. Unless you have a special reason to know something about the history of medical care, you might logically assume that it has always been under the control of uniquely qualified professionals who have spent years studying a systematic science of human health—in other words, archetypal doctors.

If you assume that doctors have always been in charge of treating illness or injury and you cannot imagine any other way of organizing a health care delivery system, you definitely need to read this chapter. Receiving medical care has not always meant "going to the doctor." In fact, going to the doctor (in today's sense of the word *doctor*) for treatment is essentially a twentieth century phenomenon. The human race has somehow managed to get through all but the last seven or eight decades of its million-year existence without granting exclusive authority over health to one professional caste. Nothing in human history or holy scripture suggests that the world will come to a screeching halt if we challenge the assumption that all health care must be provided by a doctor or someone directly supervised by a doctor. So let's challenge the assumption.

To do so, we need to understand the history behind the position taken by American doctors. Please bear with me for a quick overview of the development of medical care in general and doctors in particular. This brief review of the past helps explain why our system is as it is today—and why it can be different. Above all, it shows that medical care has been in a constant state of evolution over the past several thousand years, and there is no reason to believe that the evolution stopped for all time when doctors in the United States drummed out the competition at the beginning of this century.

Ancient Roots: Religion and Medicine

In the ancient world, the delivery of medical care was often inseparable from religion, with the role of doctor being played by priests or priestesses, medicine men, or shamans. Nevertheless, depending on the circumstance, other specialists in the healing arts were often employed. These included bone-setters, massage therapists, herbalists, exorcists, astrologers, diviners, midwives, surgeons, pharmacists, and bloodletters.[1] While the implied techniques of these "specialists" seem crude and unscientific to our modern minds, the practice of some forms of early medicine were surprisingly advanced.

---

1. Anyone who would like to learn more about the history of medicine would do well to begin with *A Short History of Medicine* (Baltimore: The Johns Hopkins University Press, 1982) by Erwin H. Ackerknecht, M.D. I have found his work to be very useful in my own teaching and writing on this fascinating subject.

For instance, as early as Neolithic Europe (roughly 5,000 to 8,000 years ago), archaeologists find evidence of a form of brain surgery called trepanation, a practice by which early "surgeons" cut a cylindrical hole in the skull. Researchers theorize that it might have been done to let evil spirits escape from inside the head. Medical explanations are equally plausible, such as alleviating pressure from the brain caused by a blow or fall. We will never know for sure why this procedure was performed, but the fact that it was done many thousands of years ago (incidentally, in several widely different corners of the earth) indicates that interventionist medicine—even if the operation was performed to release evil spirits from the mind—was alive and well with Stone Age humankind.[2]

Until 3000 B.C. and even later, priestesses were both keepers of the temples and dispensers of medical care in the civilizations of the Middle East, Egypt, and Greece.[3] In the next 2500 years, medicine reached a comparatively advanced level of practice in ancient Egypt, Mesopotamia, Peru, India, and China—still in the hands of priests and priestesses. Classical Greece (500–300 B.C.) provided the bridge between ancient, metaphysically oriented medicine and modern, scientifically oriented medicine. Unlike their predecessors, Greek physicians were not priests or holy men, but lay practitioners. In fact, they were probably the first true *physicians*, i.e., medical practitioners who addressed health problems primarily from a scientific rather than a spiritual perspective. Greek diagnosis was based on physical observation rather than religious belief. Even though Greek theories of the nature of humanity and the cosmos may seem rudimentary by today's standards, they were based on principles that led to the development of the modern scientific method on which we rely—or attempt to rely—today. Certainly one of the greatest legacies that this era gave to modern medicine was the Hippocratic Oath, attributed to Hippocrates of Cos (460–379 B.C.), that details the duties and responsibilities of physicians.

---

2. Ackerknecht, *A Short History of Medicine*, pp. 8-9.
3. Mary Chamberlain, *Old Wives Tales: Their History, Remedies, and Spells* (London: Virago Press, Ltd., 1981), p. 139.

The Hippocratic Oath and Today's Doctors

Although twentieth century doctors today take the Hippocratic Oath upon graduation from medical school, how much relevance does it really have to the everyday practice of medicine in the United States in the 1990s? The actual oath is a short but somewhat diverse document that dictates how physicians ought to behave. Some of its precepts include:

• Honor and respect one's teacher, and teach the "Art" of healing to one's own sons and one's teacher's sons "without fee or stipulation," as well as to "disciples bound by a stipulation and oath according to the law of medicine, **but to none others**" (emphasis mine).[4]

• Refuse to assist in suicide or abortion.

• Live life and practice medicine "with purity and with holiness."

• Abstain "from every voluntary act of mischief and corruption, and . . . from the seduction of females or males, of freemen and slaves."

• Maintain patient privacy.

These tenets notwithstanding, the Oath most often is summed up as follows: "Above all, do no harm."[5]

All doctors in practice in the United States today have taken the Oath, but modern medical practices obviously deviate in many ways from its precepts—doctors do not lose their licenses for performing abortions or assisting with suicide, medical school professors make nice incomes teaching the art of medicine, etc. Forces other than the dictates of Hippocrates are driving the American physician today.

4. This version of the Oath is from Ackerknecht, *A Short History of Medicine*, p. 57.
5. "I will follow that system of regimen which, according to my ability and judgment, I consider for the benefit of my patients, and abstain from whatever is deleterious and mischievous."

The Hippocratic Oath, administered only to physicians, is occasionally used to defend the unique qualifications and ultimate authority of doctors. Other health professionals are considered subservient to doctors because they are not part of the fraternity that takes this 2,400-year-old pledge. Given the substantial differences between the practice of medicine today and the obligations imposed by the original Oath, I simply do not see how being admitted to the brotherhood of Hippocrates can be used as a reason to prevent others from striving to do the same good for people in need. With proper training and other attributes of professionalism as defined in the next chapter, followers of newer clinical traditions should be allowed to diagnose and treat patients without a follower of Hippocrates looking over their shoulder . . . and charging extra for providing the supervision.

I have real difficulty with justifying the medical monopoly on the basis of unique ownership of an ancient oath that is violated on a daily basis. We, the people who need expert care, should urge doctors to either abandon or update the Oath and accept the fact that it does not define a superior status that only a doctor can attain.

The theory and practice of medicine did not appreciably advance during the Roman Empire, although Galen (130–201 A.D.), a Greek physician and surgeon who had trained on gladiators, exhibited a major influence on medical thinking until the Renaissance. However, the Roman Empire did make two significant contributions to the overall health of its people—public works projects and social administration. For example, the Romans built aqueducts supplying clean water for public fountains and baths, drained swamps in and near cities, and constructed sewer systems. They also established a form of health insurance and perhaps instituted the first experiment in socialized medicine when the Roman state began employing physicians.

The Middle Ages provided some advancements on the foundations laid by Hippocrates and Galen and their respective followers, but some medical practices of pre-classical Greece were also resurrected. Toward the end of the Roman Empire, both Christians and non-Christians began relying more and more on mysticism and religion-based healing rather than scientific study. As Christianity became the prevailing Western religion, the study of medicine retreated formally into the hands of priests—particularly monks—and the advancement of medicine from a scientific point of view came to a grinding halt. At the same time, the study of medicine began to make strides in the Arab world with the ascendancy of Islam and its expansion throughout the Mediterranean. A medical encyclopedia written by the Persian Avicenna (980–1063) became a standard throughout the Western world for centuries to come.

By the twelfth century, medical study had moved out of monasteries and into universities, although medicine and the teaching thereof were still exclusively in the hands of priests. When the Church decreed at about this time that clerics could no longer practice or teach surgery, bloodletting[6] and other surgical procedures were left to various lay practitioners, particularly barbers. As Erwin Ackernecht writes, when surgery was taken out of the hands of priests, it was left to "barbers, bath-keepers, hangmen, sow-gelders, and mountebanks and quacks of every description."[7] This tradition carried on for the better part of a millennium. In Zurich in 1790, for instance, there were only "four academic doctors, but thirty-four barber-surgeons and eight midwives." Indeed, Gioacchino Rossini's famous opera of 1815, "The Barber of Seville," is historically accurate in depicting the barber as "the family doctor."

Thus, the delivery of medicine in Europe after 1200 was divided among four types of practitioner: 1) the priest-physician who studied and taught medicine at the university; 2) the general physician (often a priest) who catered to the nobility or the well-to-do; 3) the barber and other lay surgeons who, by default, were thrust into their position; and 4) the home or village healer, including herbalists and midwives, who catered to the majority of the population. The vast majority of the latter were women, many of whom walked the fine line

---

6. Bloodletting, known formally as venesection, is the practice of intentionally removing blood from the body. It is based on a belief that the causes of illness are concentrated in the blood, so health is restored as blood is drained. Leeches have been used for this purpose for thousands of years.
7. Ackerknecht, *A Short History of Medicine*, p. 89.

between being accepted (if not respected) for their skills and being branded as witches. Although the requirement that physicians be priests began to weaken, the Church still maintained a large say in the practice of formal medicine until the Renaissance.

The Renaissance and Beyond

Just as Renaissance life reflected the upheaval in Western art and science, Renaissance medicine reflected the conflict between Church-dominated methodologies and the rediscovery of man's power to change the world. This opened up a new direction in medicine, beginning with the serious study of physical anatomy, a pursuit which had been discouraged by the Church. A new age of discovery and description was launched by thinkers like Galileo, Copernicus, Leonardo da Vinci, and others—all trying to find cause and effect in the physical world. Yet medicine as we know it was still in its infancy. Even the most progressive physicians, anatomists, and scientists believed in such things as alchemy and astrology.

The practice of surgery, still separate from the non-invasive practice of medicine by university-educated physicians, began to gain some respectability during the sixteenth century. At the same time, barber-surgeons were beginning to compete with midwives in the practice of obstetrics.[8] We in the United States are still directly affected by the results of this development—the gradual takeover of women's health and childbirth by male barber-surgeons and physicians from female nurse-midwives who, in most cultures, had been performing these duties since the dawn of humankind.

The advancements of the fifteenth and sixteenth centuries led directly to the explosion of scientific and medical knowledge in the seventeenth. The circulatory, respiratory, and lymphatic systems, as well as bacteria and cells, were all "discovered," thanks in part to the development of the compound microscope. Diseases of the day attracted significant scientific attention and were more accurately studied and described than ever before, but treatment remained elusive. University-trained physicians still had one foot in medievalism, and the practice of medicine was open to any and all who claimed that ability.[9]

---

8. Ackerknecht, *A Short History of Medicine*, p. 110.
9. Ackerknecht, *A Short History of Medicine*, p. 127.

The American Way

Until the end of the nineteenth century, medical care in North America was provided by a hodge-podge of healers with widely varying backgrounds— clerics, midwives, pharmacists, medicine men and women, and just about anybody claiming to have a cure—along with a few formally trained physicians. Being a medical school graduate in America was exceedingly rare until well into the 1800s. The study of medicine led only to an undergraduate degree, if any degree at all, and often could be accomplished with a minimum of academic study. More than likely, medicine was learned through an apprenticeship to another physician, just as midwifery was learned by working alongside an experienced midwife.

America was still predominantly a rural nation, and the criteria for giving (and receiving) medical help had more to do with location than with training. In the cities, however, there were a few formal medical practices managed by university-trained physicians.[10] While most of our nation's early doctors came from Europe, more and more were educated in this country once the first medical school was established in Philadelphia in 1765. Some attempts to organize and even license physicians were made in the more populated states in the late 1700s, but the efforts floundered.

The state of American medicine remained disorganized until the mid-nineteenth century—a direct reflection of the *laissez-faire* policies of Jacksonian democracy (named after Andrew Jackson, who was elected in the 1820s and 1830s on a campaign platform that shunned government regulation of almost any kind) and the country's rapid expansion west. In 1846, a group of physicians banded together to form what was to become the American Medical Association—the AMA—but its early impact on medical care was minimal. Not only did those who called themselves "doctors" remain divided and intensely competitive in their individual approaches, but they also competed with the many lay practitioners—mostly women—who delivered much of the medical care of the day.

---

10. Two excellent books are recommended to the reader who would like to study the development of American medicine in more detail: Rosemary Stevens' *American Medicine and the Public Interest* (New Haven: Yale University Press, 1971); and Paul Starr's *The Social Transformation of American Medicine* (New York: Basic Books, 1982).

A few key developments during the nineteenth century served to advance medical science and thereby turn medicine into a learned profession. (We need to remember that bloodletting and purging, the evacuation of the system by stimulating the bowels, were still primary treatments for a host of ailments well into the 1800s.) Advancements such as vaccinations, anesthesia, and the use of antiseptics and sterile surgical procedures all contributed to the definition of modern medicine in the mid- to late 1800s. Louis Pasteur's discovery of the microbial cause of infectious disease did not occur until 1864. Prior to this remarkable advancement, health providers had no definitive understanding of the physical mechanisms that led to illness, nor could they prove any cause-and-effect relationship between their care and changes in their patients' health.

Many "medical schools" proliferated in late nineteenth century America, espousing a host of philosophical approaches to diagnosis and treatment. These schools bore little resemblance to the high-quality medical training institutions that we have today. They were more like trade or technical schools, with students gaining admission upon completing the equivalent of high school. The schools offered as little as three or four months to a year of basic courses, which were often repeated for a second year. Although many of these schools were attached to general colleges or universities, students commonly paid their tuition directly to the professors—usually doctors needing a little extra income. The students were expected to go on to apprenticeship training after the classroom instruction, although this applied learning did not always happen.

Given this disorganized general state of affairs—and the low incomes that resulted from such a highly competitive market where virtually anyone could be a doctor—organized medical societies like the AMA began pushing states toward setting basic standards for physician licensing. This movement began in the 1870s, but the United States Supreme Court did not officially recognize the right of states to license doctors until 1888. Giving states the power to restrict who could be a doctor was the first step toward giving medical doctors the monopoly they enjoy today. Within 30 years, every state had some sort of medical licensing law.

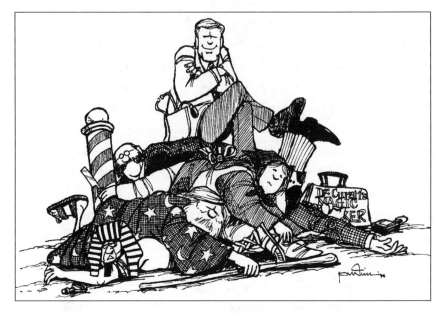

While licensing physicians did serve to protect the public from "diploma mill" quacks and charlatans, it also placed the control of who could and could not practice medicine into the hands of the university-trained physicians. These doctors gained not only the power to police themselves, but also the power to establish the new order of medical care in the United States (giving one meaning to the title of this book, i.e., creating order according to doctors' wishes). The "losers" were not just bogus or poorly trained doctors, but experienced lay practitioners such as midwives who were, because they were women or ethnic minorities, all but excluded from the form of higher education dominated by white males. In fact, one of the AMA's early positions was to oppose the "ignorant meddlesome midwife," both as an abortionist and a caregiver.[11]

Despite this consolidation of control by the medical profession, the many medical schools that had proliferated across the country during the latter part of the nineteenth century were only loosely regulated. The AMA, which had reorganized and was now quickly growing to represent over half of the physicians in the country, commissioned Abraham Flexner of the Carnegie Foundation in 1908 to examine all the medical schools in the country. His report, released in 1910, condemned all but a handful of schools as being substandard. While

---

11. See Susan Faludi, *Backlash: The Undeclared War Against American Women* (New York: Crown, 1991), p. 413, and The Boston Women's Health Book Collective, *The New Our Bodies, Ourselves*, 1992 edition (New York: Touchstone, 1992), p. 692.

many schools were already in a weakened condition due to the new licensing laws and other changes in the medical profession, the Flexner Report thrust medical education into a period of reform and consolidation—firmly under control of the AMA. Within five years, the number of medical schools in the country dropped by one-third, from 131 to 95.[12] By the mid-1920s, that number had dwindled even further. Only a few dozen medical schools remained to train the kind of doctor with the professional stamp of approval. Competition was neutralized in the name of educational reform.

This consolidation served to homogenize medical education into an institution of, by, and for upper-class white males. It also served to define doctors who met that criterion as the sole source of medical care in the country. In the process, five of the seven black medical schools closed, as well as two out of the three medical schools established for women. In the schools that did survive, no more than 5 percent of the student positions were allocated to women.[13]

The philosophical thrust of the revamped medical schools was even more limiting. As Rocio Huet-Cox writes:

> The Flexner Report served, in essence, to establish a highly durable model for medicine—disease-oriented and mechanistic, centrally based in the hospital or office, and focused on the individual patient. In this model, the sick or injured individual comes to the solo practitioner for a rational assessment of an illness. The physician then attempts to "cure" the patient with the diagnostic and therapeutic tools placed at his disposal by biomedical research and technology.[14]

Medical schools, and thus doctors, came to embody the *allopathic* approach to medicine—that is, there is no need for intervention until a problem occurs, whereupon it is dealt with in a systematic and scientific way.

Other philosophical approaches did not immediately disappear. However, some alternative views of disease and treatment that had gained strength in the latter part of the nineteenth century gradually faded away (see sidebar: "Homeopathy and Eclecticism"). Others—most notably osteopathy, chiro-

---

12. Starr, *The Social Transformation of American Medicine*, p. 120.
13. Starr, *The Social Transformation of American Medicine*, p. 124.
14. Victor W. Sidell and Ruth Sidell (eds.), *Reforming Medicine: Lessons of the Last Quarter Century* (New York: Pantheon Books, 1984), p. 131.

practic, and Christian Science—survived on the fringes of the professionally approved model, allopathic medicine. Christian Science sought refuge in religious practice and gained immunity from the secular laws of the several states, while osteopathy and chiropractic managed to survive as professionally disputed alternatives to the allopathic physician.

Homeopathy and Eclecticism

Two of the more prominent alternatives coexisting with mainstream medicine during the latter half of the nineteenth century were offered by the homeopaths and the eclectics. The latter served mainly to oppose some of the aggressive treatments of the day such as bloodletting, purging, vomiting, and toxic drug therapy. Instead of accepting these therapies, eclectics took their course of treatment from herbalism as much as mainstream scientific medicine.

The homeopaths advocated treating disease by injecting minute quantities of natural, symptom-producing substances into the patient—substances that were known to cause the same or similar symptoms as the disease. As a widely accepted form of medical practice, it quickly lost favor within the first two decades of the twentieth century, arguably because of the offensive of licensing and educational reforms launched by mainstream scientific medicine.[15] Nevertheless, it still survives today as a "fringe" medicine in the United States; homeopathy is more widely accepted in Europe. For example, in France homeopaths are reimbursed as regular practitioners by the health insurance system.

15. Paul Starr claims both eclecticism and homeopathy were absorbed into mainstream allopathic medicine, rather than shunned by it. Presumably, eclecticism lost some of its thrust as mainstream cures grew more humane, and homeopathy, without a firm scientific base, simply could no longer attract students. A parallel today might be drawn to osteopathic medicine, which for many years opposed allopathy, but today is all but part of it. (See Starr, *The Social Transformation of American Medicine*, pp. 107-08.)

In many areas of the United States, osteopathic medicine is now considered as acceptable as allopathic medicine. Allopaths and osteopaths are both defined as physicians in state medical practice acts, with the same privileges and scopes of practice. Both attend four years of medical school and take the same examinations to become licensed. Doctors of both types commonly practice together without any ill feelings toward one another. However, I have recently been in parts of the Midwest where doctors and patients alike are deeply divided over the presumed differences between osteopathy and allopathy (see sidebar: "Allopathy and Osteopathy"). The bitter divisions of the late nineteenth century are still present in some areas!

Allopathy and Osteopathy

Allopathy, the clinical foundation of mainstream American medicine since the educational reforms of the early twentieth century, is based on the belief that the physician's role is to create within the patient a physical environment to fight the diagnosed illness or injury. Consequently, allopathic physicians use active and invasive interventions, such as drugs and surgery, to counteract the factors that are believed to cause disease. Physicians who graduate from an allopathic medical school are designated by the M.D. degree.

Osteopathy is based on the same conceptual foundations as allopathy, but it additionally emphasizes the relationship between organs and the musculoskeletal system. Therefore, like chiropractors and unlike allopaths, osteopaths use manipulation as part of their approach to healing. Physicians who graduate from a college of osteopathic medicine receive the D.O. degree.

The treatment of nursing was particularly interesting. Nurses were declared "the doctors' handmaidens" and removed from any further consideration of independent practice. The assumption was that nurses could not exist without doctors, and that was that. Nursing's only bright spot in the formative years of the medical care system came when Florence Nightingale pioneered the concept of the "clean" hospital during the Crimean War. Despite this innovation, which saved countless lives and transformed the hospital from a place where people died to a place where people regained health, her accomplishments on behalf of nursing never elevated the profession above the doctor-subservient role it has played ever since.

The Golden Age of American Medicine: The 1920s to the 1960s

By 1920, the allopathic doctor was firmly in the driver's seat of American medicine. Competing philosophies such as homeopathy and eclecticism had either joined up or left town, nonphysician providers had been placed in a subservient role, and lay practitioners had been conveniently shoved into the closet. Within just a few decades, medicine had gone from a totally unregulated situation to a highly advanced state of regulation under the control of the order of allopathic doctors (that is, the AMA). The state medical practice acts had defined the practice of medicine, then limited that practice only to individuals who had graduated from medical schools accredited according to the standards of the university-trained practitioners. Though the specific details of the medical practice acts varied from state to state—for example, some states required an internship or residency before a physician could be licensed, some did not—their impact was basically the same: they placed the practice of medicine entirely into the hands of the allopathic doctors. The AMA, which in the mid-1800s was one struggling medical society among many, came to control the decision-making process of American medicine by the early 1900s.

Not that other practitioners were ignored . . . states also began passing acts to regulate the practice of nonphysician medical occupations such as nursing, physical therapy, occupational therapy, laboratory technology, and pharmacy. These professional practice acts were carefully written so as not to encroach on the doctors' ultimate authority. In some states, the authority for many of these other providers is still contained within the medical practice act, leaving no doubt who is in control. As will be shown in the next chapter, the doctor was able to gain control of all potential competitors by retaining the authority of "captain of the ship."

But the doctors' authority was not without challenge. Socialized medical insurance had already begun in Europe, and attempts were made in this country to promote various forms of practice that placed the physician in the position of being an employee of (and thus subservient to) a larger organization such as a corporation or a fraternal order. Furthermore, hospitals were growing both in stature and economic clout, and indemnity insurance was gaining in acceptance. The official party line of organized medicine was that the doctor should remain free and independent of all outside authority (i.e., financial considerations should not enter into the selection of optimal treatment), should work only on a fee-for-service basis, and should protect at all costs the sanctity of the relationship between himself and his patient.

The state medical practice acts provided the framework for doctors' responses to these challenges to their professional authority. The laws were written at the behest of the physician—allowing doctors to determine the rules of medical practice rather than giving government the power to write guidelines for them. Doctors made sure they were the only ones who sat on state licensing boards and medical review panels. When the laws needed to be changed, doctors drafted the changes for the legislators to adopt. When regulations needed to be written for other health care providers and for hospitals, doctors took care of that task, too.

This situation contrasts significantly with the standard approach to regulated public utilities. In virtually every case but medical practice, the regulatory body consisted of outsiders appointed by the government. In the case of medicine, doctors secured the power to regulate themselves under the guise of being a learned profession—one so special that outsiders could not possibly know enough to regulate in the public interest. A classic case of putting the fox in charge of the chicken coop.

The same professional autonomy was preserved in the case of medical insurance. As noted previously, doctors fought strenuously in the 1920s and 1930s against the concept of third-party coverage on the grounds that it intruded on the doctor-patient relationship. But realizing that "the best way to beat 'em is to join 'em," doctors deflected the threatened loss of control by establishing Blue Cross (for hospital-based treatment) and Blue Shield (for physicians' services). Again, organized medicine worked the legislatures to secure special treatment for its insurance plan—nonprofit status and exemption from insurance laws that required control by outside directors. With special treatment like this, the physician-controlled "Blues" were able to corner the market on health insurance, too.

The periodic push for socialized medicine likewise provided a challenge for the doctors. Teddy Roosevelt proposed government-controlled health insurance in 1912 as the Progressive Party candidate for President. It again was raised as part of the New Deal legislation during the 1930s, but opposition by physicians ultimately caused it to be left out of the Social Security Act. The issue arose again during both the Truman and Nixon presidencies, only to be branded as "socialism" by the AMA and other groups with a vested interest in the status quo.[16] The doctors' independence and their authority over the American medical care system remained intact. Indeed, this power had become so strong that *the doctor had broadened his fiefdom to cover the entire health care system, blurring the division between medical care and health care and minimizing the importance of public health and preventive medicine.* Of course, staying in control is a lot easier when you don't have any competition.

Physicians did not meet their match until Lyndon Johnson became President in 1963 following the assassination of John F. Kennedy. A Democratic Congress and a strong Democratic president combined forces to create Medicare and Medicaid, programs designed to provide health services to the nation's elderly and the poor who were covered by Social Security. Doctors, of course, vigorously fought Medicare and Medicaid for the usual reasons: the threat of socialized medicine and government interference with the doctor-

---

16. For those too young to remember Senator Joe McCarthy and the Cold War, anything considered un-American by defenders of the *status quo* was labeled "socialistic" or, even worse, "communistic." These labels were strongly pejorative, often used to suggest that people who would propose such new ideas were unpatriotic "sympathizers" trying to overthrow the U.S. government. I can vividly remember respected doctors labeling the health maintenance organization concept as a "communist plot" when I was doing research on it in 1973! The era was not kind to progressive thinkers.

patient relationship. The compromise leading to passage in 1965 was designation of "the Blues"—still controlled by the physicians—as administrators of the Medicare plan. Doctors were bruised but not beaten, and before long they learned that this new infusion of federal money into "their system" turned charity patients without any insurance into paying patients with government insurance—leading doctors on an unprecedented journey of higher incomes, increased social status, and guaranteed employment.

In economic theory, competition from acceptable nonphysician providers would have led to a more equitable distribution of income. In practice, however, physicians were still "the only game in town." When people wanted health care as recently as 1965, no one but a doctor was sufficiently qualified to provide it. However, doctors' rapid acceptance of Medicare and Medicaid unwittingly and ironically led them to create the new professionals who are now qualified to bring competitive efficiency to the medical marketplace. Read on.

Beyond the Fein Line

In 1967, two years after the enactment of Medicare and Medicaid, Harvard economist Rashi Fein published *The Doctor Shortage*,[17] a book that projected that the United States would face a severe shortage of doctors by the mid-1980s. The book bore the imprint of the prestigious Brookings Institution and received a great deal of attention during the last year of the Johnson Administration's social idealism. The book's impact on medical thinking was not unlike the impact of Michael Harrington's *The Other America*[18] on the social thinking that created many antipoverty programs of President Lyndon B. Johnson's Great Society.

Congress responded to Fein's book in the late 1960s and early 1970s by passing several National Health Manpower Development Acts, which formally established a national policy objective of doubling the number of physicians in practice by 1985. This goal would be accomplished by making unprecedented sums available to states to expand existing medical schools and to establish new ones. Medicare and Medicaid were obviously going to increase

17. Rashi Fein, *The Doctor Shortage: An Economic Diagnosis*, (Washington D.C.: Brookings Institution), 1967.
18. Michael Harrington, *The Other America* (New York: Viking Penguin, 1971).

the demand for medical care, so preventing the predicted doctor shortage became one of the nation's top social priorities.

Because of the fear that our country would not be able to increase the number of doctors fast enough, other health professions volunteered to help. In particular, dentistry and nursing jumped on the bandwagon and began to expand their respective roles in patient care. New training programs proliferated throughout the 1970s and early 1980s. Federal money was readily available for any accredited academic health center that wanted to join the campaign to overcome the doctor shortage predicted by Professor Fein. Two generic terms were developed to describe the more than 100 different categories of non-physician providers: "allied health providers" and "physician extenders."[19] Programs were started to educate not only more physicians, but many new health professionals as well.

Within a few years, allied health providers and physician extenders were ready to take over some of the doctors' traditional tasks. Feeling secure in their status and fearing shortage-induced overwork, physicians were willing to let this happen for the first time since passage of the state medical practice acts. The medical profession as a whole was on a roll, fueled by a combination of the perceived doctor shortage, social idealism, the country's willingness and ability to spend money on health care, and the very real increases in demand created by Medicare and Medicaid.

Meanwhile, other factors were influencing the nursing profession—the largest, if not the most influential, of the allied health professions. Driven by both the growing feminist movement and economic necessity, more and more young women were choosing a career over the traditional housewife role. Many women who wanted to enter the medical field saw nursing as a logical choice. On the practical side, nursing education was a much less drastic commitment than medical school. But more importantly—at a time when the professional equality of the sexes was still a relatively new concept—nursing was, after all, a "woman's profession" (see sidebar: "The Nursing Model").

---

19. The programs were growing faster than we could catalog them. I served as recording secretary to the American Association of Academic Health Center's national committee on allied health-training programs during the early 1980s; our list of new job classifications grew at every meeting, and we never did feel the list was up to date.

The Nursing Model

The nursing model is quite different from that of allopathic physicians, which means that nurses and doctors do not always share the same concepts of patient care. While the allopathic physician model is aggressive, invasive, and symptom-oriented (i.e., "Let's look at the disease"), the nursing model puts considerably more direct emphasis on the patient's mental, physical, and emotional well-being. Nurses' training emphasizes personal contact, listening, and caring—in short, a more holistic approach. The difference is sometimes summed up in the aphorism: Doctors look at the chart, nurses see the patient.

Some medical theorists have argued that the doctor model is inherently "masculine" and the nursing model "feminine," the doctor model "active" and the nursing model "passive," etc. Certainly, a highly sexist division of labor is consistent with medicine's exclusion of women at the beginning of the twentieth century. Of course, the medical model might be different in the future now that half of all students admitted to medical school are women.

Enrollments in nursing programs began to swell in the 1970s. Up to this time, the vast majority of nurses had gone through two-year or three-year diploma programs that were more apprenticeship than academic in nature. Most of these programs were hospital-based and administered under the tutelage of doctors. Completion of the program offered not a college degree, but a diploma usually conferred in a "capping ceremony" by (who else?) a doctor. The role of the nurse was still what it had been for over a century—to be the "doctor's handmaiden."

However, the massive infusion of federal funds for health education fueled an unexpected revolution in nursing. Doctors may have controlled the hospital-based diploma programs, but they did not control the schools of nursing within state and private universities. Academic leaders in the nursing profession began to push for full four-year nursing programs leading to a bachelor's degree.[20] Even M.S. and Ph.D. degrees in nursing became widely available for the first time in the late 1970s. Nursing education experienced renewal comparable to the turn-of-the-century reforms of medical education. In particular, nursing also adopted four years of university training as the standard for entry into practice.

The enhancement of nursing education was initially done with the tacit blessing of doctors who readily acknowledged the need for more and better trained nurses. However, doctors were undoubtedly expecting the nursing schools to train more "doctor's handmaidens," not professional nurses qualified for independent practice. Aghast at what it had allowed to happen, in the early 1990s the AMA proposed to establish its own programs to train the kind of nurse-technicians who followed doctors' orders. The plan received no support outside the medical profession and was quietly withdrawn in mid-1993 as the AMA had to turn its attention to the battle over health reform. The failure of this effort to put nursing back in its traditional place may mark the end of the unique reign of doctors—"not with a bang, but a whimper."[21]

While federal health policy was preparing for a domestic crisis in medical care delivery, the Vietnam War was creating its own demand for health care professionals. The doctor shortage was even more acute in the military because of medical student deferments and lack of volunteer enlistments for an unpopular war where doctors on the front line faced a 50-50 chance of coming home in a box. As a result, the military began to train its own medics and corpsmen in many medical skills, including some complex procedures (e.g., restoring airways, removing ruptured appendixes, stabilizing erratic heart rhythms) that had previously been performed only by doctors.

The stateside return of these military-trained medics after the war created a new stress on the system. Many had little more than a high school education, yet they had been trained—and trained well—to do many things that only doctors did before. The physician's assistant (PA) movement was the result.

---

20. I served for several years in the late 1970s as the planning consultant to the Roles and Functions Committee of the American Nurses Association. I remember very well the incredible enthusiasm for defining the background and skills of the professional nurse. Many of the educational reforms in nursing schools during the 1980s were a direct result of the extensive work done by this committee.
21. T.S. Eliot, "The Wasteland."

Several medical schools and other health sciences institutions began to train civilians (many of whom were former medics or corpsmen using their veterans' educational benefits) to perform a number of advanced procedures as PAs, provided they worked under a doctor's supervision.

Even more competition for the medical profession was created when Congress passed several National Highway Transportation Safety Acts in the late 1960s and 1970s. These laws set up a system of emergency medical technicians and paramedics trained specifically for emergency pre-hospital care of seriously injured patients. Until this system was established, most private ambulance services were operated by mortuaries—a rather morbid conflict of interest by today's standards. The creation of emergency medical services (EMS) systems provided the newly trained professionals with the skills to stabilize critical patients at the scene before transporting them to definitive medical care, a real life-saving improvement over the "scoop-and-run" approach that prevailed before creation of the EMS system. Paramedics have proven that someone besides a doctor can save a life.

At approximately the same time, a well-known pediatrician named Henry Silver (my colleague at the University of Colorado School of Medicine; we had adjacent offices, so some of his thinking must have passed through the wall) decided that nurses could be trained to provide most pediatric care in a fully professional and competent manner. After all, the vast majority of nurses were women, and many were mothers; they knew what kids were like. Dr. Silver also saw no direct correlation between physicians' residency training for pediatrics—three years of caring for high-risk infants in a large teaching hospital— and the most common pediatric duties, such as dealing with ear aches and giving routine physicals. He saw the situation as a classic misallocation of resources and created the nation's first Child Health Associate Program to train nonphysician pediatric health care specialists. He also went to the Colorado legislature and, for the first time since the creation of the state medical practice acts, secured legal authority for these new nonphysician providers to diagnose and treat patients without the supervision of a physician.

Nursing schools also began offering advanced training leading to a master's degree in basic nursing skills. Many of the graduates from these new, graduate-level programs became nurse practitioners. Though trained to diagnose and treat a number of illnesses from the perspective of the nursing model, advanced practice nurses often found themselves limited by the state medical practice acts. They had at least as much training as physicians in a broad base of primary health services, but they had to work under the umbrella (and fee structure) of a physician.

Finally, as a late-1970s concession to meeting the needs of Medicare and Medicaid patients, nurse practitioners and other new providers began to win the right to practice independently of physicians in a few states. Open-minded legislators in these states finally began asking the same questions that had been asked by the growing numbers of new, well-trained professionals, "Why is the practice of medicine in this country reserved only to doctors? We can provide many of these services, perform many of these tasks, just as well, if not better. Why can't we be allowed to do the jobs we're trained to do?" The doctors' economically self-serving answers were no longer convincing.

As this historical review has shown, the national response to the impending doctor shortage was moving full-speed ahead by the mid-1970s. For a variety of reasons, its progress was not being controlled by organized medicine. By the early 1980s, a few states began loosening the power of medical practice acts and allowing some nonphysician providers to practice independently of doctors. On the theory of "better late than never," the mid-1990s would be an ideal time to incorporate the state-level successes with independent nonphysician providers into national health policy. (President Clinton's administration deserves credit for including this general concept in its overall health reform proposal. Under the direction of Hillary Rodham Clinton, the White House Task Force on Health Reform devoted considerable effort to exploring the issue. Sadly, its efforts to promote nonphysician providers are obscured by the "rube goldberg"[22] nature of the rest of the Clinton plan.) Real health reform will take advantage of the availability of these qualified professionals who can compete with doctors. Anything less will be a tragically missed opportunity to do something meaningful about the medical monopoly.

---

22. Reuben L. Goldberg was an early twentieth century American cartoonist known for his detailed drawing of unnecessarily complicated, overdesigned devices for doing simple things.

Beyond the Doctor Shortage

1983 was a watershed year in health care finance. Prior to 1983, almost all reimbursement—meaning third-party insurance—was paid to hospitals on a retrospective, cost-based system. Hospitals would bill the public and private insurers according to the cost of providing service as determined after the service was incurred. The insurers sent back the requested amount as payment, no questions asked. Then, in 1983, Congress unexpectedly passed legislation to create a *prospective* payment system (PPS) for Medicare reimbursements to hospitals. This dramatic change in federal health policy was basically an expression of congressional disgust with the uncontrolled growth in medical spending that was being largely financed by the American taxpayer, while doctors and hospitals were making out like bandits. The providers did not have to make any long-term sacrifices in cost containment because the federal government had developed a payment policy that amounted to writing blank checks.

The prospective payment system was Congress' way of fixing the size of the health care "pie" by determining in advance exactly how much the federal government was willing to spend on health care (in contrast to the retrospective system that paid whatever the providers charged). Reimbursement was further simplified by lumping thousands of hospital-based procedures into a few hundred diagnostic related groups, or DRGs. The same general reimbursement method was later applied to payments to physicians under the acronym RBRVS (Resource-Based Relative Value System, euphemistically known to doctors before its implementation in 1992 as Really Bad Reimbursement Very Soon).

Congress went after hospitals first because they accounted for roughly 40 percent of all health care dollars spent, roughly twice the level of spending on physicians' services. After successfully forcing a new payment system on hospitals (which was not necessarily the same as successfully reducing hospital expenditures), Congress decided to go after the doctors. In the late 1980s, a Harvard economist named William Hsiao was commissioned to develop a physician reimbursement system that reflected the actual cost of providing services rather than historical charges that did not necessarily reflect true costs of production.[23]

Doctors were used to being reimbursed on the basis of "usual, customary, and reasonable" (UCR) fees. Insurers looked at the profile of all fees for a particular service or procedure and paid any submitted fee up to a certain cut-off point—commonly the 90th percentile. This system may be noteworthy for refusing to pay the "unreasonable" fees in the top 10 percent, but it did not reflect any competition in the marketplace. Nothing in the system prevented a constant general rise in the overall fee profile. For example, new physicians would look around to see what other physicians were charging and select fees near the top, which raised the overall average. Insurance companies, led by the doctor-controlled "Blues" and dependent upon the physician for business, would unquestioningly pay the submitted fees, with the token rejection of the highest charges. A truly competitive market would never support such a nice financial arrangement. Doctors, with no outside competition, could charge more or less whatever they wanted and be confident that they would be reimbursed for a healthy portion of their bills.

Even though the Hsiao study was generated by a policy of bringing reimbursement in line with actual costs—something the UCR system did not do— it was conducted in a highly political environment and has been criticized for resulting methodological flaws. (Even Professor Hsiao himself has expressed dismay at what has been done with the results of his study.[24]) Further, RBRVS has not lived up to its other attempt at fairness. In addition to bringing fees in line with actual costs, the system was also supposed to transfer some income from highly paid proceduralists, i.e., surgeons, to the cognitive doctors, i.e., noninvasive primary-care physicians, whose services had presumably been undervalued by surgeon-controlled insurance companies. (Why, I've always wondered, would the second focus on redistribution even be necessary if the RBRVS study produced accurate cost-based fees for all groups of physicians? Must have something to do with politics!)

---

23. Hsiao, W.C. et al., "Estimating Physician's Work for a Resource-Based Relative Value Scale," *New England Journal of Medicine 319:835-41(1988)*.
24. Hsiao, W.C. et al., "Assessing the Implementation of Physician Payment Reform," *New England Journal of Medicine 328:928-33(1993)*.

If This Makes Sense, You Don't Understand . . .

The DRG reimbursement system was based on a health care quality model developed by a Yale professor, John Thompson. His model had nothing to do with payment systems, but his research was being widely discussed when the government was looking for a new way to structure payment. The bureaucracy appropriated his quality assessment model and tried to make it fit the payment system, which probably helps explain why the PPS failed to stop the increases in hospital spending. Worse yet, historical costs were used as the basis for DRG payments. No analysis of actual cost was ever performed, so the whole system just repackages the inefficiencies of cost-based reimbursement.

In my opinion, if you've read all about DRGs and the prospective payment system, gone to all the courses and spent hours trying to understand them, and they still don't make sense to you, you understand DRGs. On the other hand, if you think that the DRG system is logical and easy to understand, you don't know what's going on. It's a nonsense system. It's like something out of Alice in Wonderland.

Public pronouncements to the contrary, most members of Congress really do not care whether the prospective payment system is fair or not. Many elected officials believed when voting for the change that doctors and hospitals had taken advantage of the Medicare system, then nearly 20 years old. The intent of the prospective payment system was to give patients better access to health care and to end the rapidly increasing and unpredictable expenditures on government-funded health care. Regardless of the economic wisdom (or lack thereof) in the DRG and RBRVS payment mechanisms, creation of the prospective payment system 10 years ago does indicate that the medical care delivery system is no longer under the control of providers. Washington ought to be receptive to the idea of freeing qualified competitors from following doctors' orders.

By learning how to bill for the DRG that was most profitable, a practice known as "gaming the system," hospitals quickly and legally discovered ways to make money on DRGs. A whole industry of reimbursement consultants has been created to stay one step ahead of changes in the government's payment regulations—an expected development that makes an intelligent observer question the wisdom of basing health care reform on modifications of the payment system. Today's real savings in hospital expenditures can be traced to competition from outpatient services and productivity-enhancing technology, not the 1983-based changes in reimbursement methodology.

We need to harness the government's willingness to challenge providers and redirect it from payment reform to provider reform—beginning with laws that open up the practice of medicine to qualified nonphysician providers. At present, doctors in the United States are enjoying monopoly incomes that result from the protection of state medical practice acts. Nowhere else in the world has government allowed the medical profession to manage itself and to set its own fees. In the process of our national mobilization to head off the doctor shortage, we created a solution far better than regulation. *It's called competition, and its time has come.*

Into the Twenty-First Century

The basic principles of chaos theory may be the best tools for looking at American medicine today. The old structure is crumbling. Doctors are becoming disenchanted with the practice of medicine. The rules are changing fast. The paperwork is awesome—in the last 10 years, the number of billing clerks per physician in private practice has gone from one-and-a-half to four. (This is not because of more patients; it is simply because of more paperwork.) The result is that the vast majority of new doctors finishing medical training are choosing to work for someone else rather than setting up a private practice. We see rapid growth in larger health care organizations where employed doctors work on salary, a major change from the historic fee-for-service system.

Health care has become highly politicized, too. The state medical practice acts were the first government intrusion into the practice of medicine. These laws were 100 percent friendly to the allopathic doctor—justifiably eliminating competitors who kept incomes low while having no proof of the value of their treatments. For more than half a century, university-trained doctors labored mightily and successfully to preserve their control over all the delivery of medical care. The beginning of the end of the golden age of American medicine came in 1965 when government became a major purchaser of health services via Medicare and Medicaid. Then, by accepting the proposed solutions to the predicted manpower shortage, doctors allowed other health professionals to achieve the qualifications for independent practice.

Mrs. Thiam, Friendly Neighborhood Kidney Doctor

When I was a student in Geneva, Switzerland, in the early 1970s, I had a room in a condemned building that looked nice on the outside, but it had bad plumbing on the inside. That's why it was condemned. I lived on one end of a hallway. On the opposite end of the hallway was a nephrologist—a kidney specialist—on the staff of the local hospital.

She was a very nice lady and dedicated doctor. But she was living in the same condemned building as me because she did not make enough money to live at a fancy address. As a nephrologist she was highly respected. Yet as a human being—as a professional providing a valuable service to society—she was treated like you and me and everybody else. She didn't have any monopoly power.

This experience and extensive foreign travel have shown me that doctors in most other countries of the world don't possess the special economic power they receive in the United States. Yet they are just as committed to their patients. Good, even great, people can be attracted to the practice of medicine by benefits other than high incomes.

Mysteriously, the obvious implications of this last change have been over-looked thus far in the public debate over health reform. The President, the Congress, and many state legislatures are all convinced that now is the time to make big changes. Sadly, their approach is keyed to one question: "How else should we pay the doctor?" The real question ought to be, "Who in addition to the doctor ought to be paid?" The American public and the politicians need to go beyond the issue of payment reform and physician regulation, both of which play into the hands of the medical monopoly. The American public needs to ask itself and its leaders, "What is the most efficient way to provide quality health care to the country?" The answer will be following something other than doctors' orders.

Chapter Four

Captain of the Ship

The public interest arguably was served well when many nonphysician providers of medical care were drummed out of the market in the early years of the twentieth century. In light of glaring deficiencies in the clinical knowledge and skills of these early nonphysician providers, the reformers of that era built respectable foundations for the medical monopoly we know today.

However, a new breed of qualified nonphysicians has been created over the past 25 years. Doctors no longer deserve the power to hide behind any explicit or implicit professional exemptions from antitrust law. The century-old precedent of a protected monopoly, one that effectively allows physicians to prevent other qualified sellers from entering "their" marketplace, is not in the public interest as we move toward the twenty-first century. We must break up the established order.

To their enduring credit, turn-of-the century physicians did not evade the professional responsibilities of newfound power. While their motivations for eliminating competition may have been economically self-serving, the founders of the medical monopoly were truly dedicated to the integrity of medical practice. These medical reformers believed in the Hippocratic dictates that doctors should heal themselves and do no harm. They performed a service by protecting the public from competitors whose treatments (e.g., leeches, poisonous nostrums) were often worse than the diseases they sought to cure.

Turn-of-the-century physicians in the United States did not deserve to be ranked with their industrial contemporaries, the robber barons, who cared not at all about protecting consumers in markets managed under the principle of "buyer beware." Medical doctors' primary concern in the early twentieth century was the welfare of their patients. At a time when many of their non-physician competitors cared more about making an income than providing safe and appropriate services, scientifically based physicians of that era deserved to be given sole authority as "captain of the ship."

The **"captain of the ship" doctrine** is the legal principle of placing the medical doctor at the top of the medical care hierarchy and making all other health care providers subject to his orders. *In return for this authority, the physician accepts all responsibility and accountability for the care of the patient.* The doctrine gives the physician ultimate, final control over all medical decision making. In other words, just as the captain of a seagoing vessel has ultimate authority and responsibility over the entire crew, everyone on the health care team—nurse, pharmacist, therapist, aide—reports to the doctor.

Anyone seeking medical care can readily see the extent of the doctor's authority, as illustrated by three scenarios of everyday medical care.

Scenario 1: A clinic nurse greets a mother and her child with an earache and ushers them to an examination room down a hall. She takes the child's temperature and asks a few questions. When she's done, she instructs the mother to wait for the doctor, who inevitably is "running a little bit late, but will be here as soon as he can." Twenty minutes later, the doctor arrives. The child has since fallen asleep, giving the mother her first bit of quiet time since the evening before. The physician awakens the child, performs the examination, makes the diagnosis, and writes out the prescription. The examination takes less than five minutes and he is gone, leaving the mother with a piece of paper and a fussy child once more. Under the "captain of the ship" doctrine it makes no difference that a nurse practitioner, who has received the same training in how to diagnose and treat an ear infection, could have completed the examination much sooner and at less expense.

Scenario 2: An old man lies in a hospital bed recovering from a bout of pneumonia. The nurse by his bedside encourages him to take his pills, but he refuses. He doesn't like to swallow them. "It hurts," he says. She's heard this before. She knows that she would have more luck giving him the medicine in liquid form, but the written instructions from the physician, who has only visited the man twice, expressly state he is to receive pills. Regardless of her education or experience, she has no authority to make a change (see sidebar: "Lillian").

Scenario 3: A woman who is newly arrived in town hands a young pharmacist a prescription for her asthmatic teenage son. "It's different from what we've been taking," she says, "but we'll give it a try." The pharmacist knows the drug well. The general practitioner whose name is on the slip has been prescribing this same drug for the last 10 years despite ample literature indicating more effective alternatives, some at a lower cost. But the pharmacist has no choice; she must fill the prescription as written, regardless of her superior and more recent training in pharmacology, because this particular physician does not welcome suggestions from pharmacists.

Lillian

"I was in the hospital and my temperature shot up to 102. Suddenly, here comes the rescue squad. And everyone had a job to do. They were taking blood or taking my temperature. They worked for an hour trying to get my temperature down."

"I was getting tired and wanted to go to sleep. I knew what was going on, so I said, 'I know how to get my temperature down.' They looked at me, so I said, 'Put my feet in a bucket of ice water.'"

"They looked at each other and finally a nurse said, 'We can't do that.'"

"And I said, 'Why not?'"

"The nurse said, 'Because the doctor hasn't approved it.'"

Lillian H., 77 years old

Physical therapists, occupational therapists, and speech therapists in most states have likewise been locked into providing treatment only as authorized by a physician. In many cases, these health care professionals are better trained in their fields than the doctor who issues their orders. Yet they must do the doctor's bidding, often without question, because the doctor mans the bridge. The patient is usually left out of the loop. Too often, the physician has neither the time nor the training to determine the patient's preferences. Likewise, the patient is denied the benefits of satisfaction from a knowledge-able nonphysician therapist whose hands are tied by the physician's orders.

Today, Americans give little thought to the "captain of the ship" doctrine. We find it perfectly normal that the doctor issues the orders and all other health care practitioners follow them. It is the way our medical system operates. Unless we have traveled extensively or lived abroad, it is the only system we know. And why should we complain? The doctrine has, at least indirectly, led to many of the medical advances that uniquely define American medicine, particularly high-technology interventionist medicine. Doesn't the United States have more hospital beds, more high-tech imaging machines, more operating rooms per capita than any other country in the world? Doesn't the United States provide the most advanced care in the world for those in need of bodily repair?

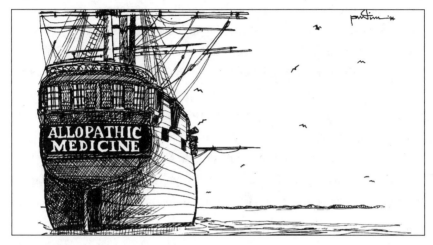

Absolutely. Because the doctor has been the captain of the American medical ship for most of this century, our health care delivery system has been tailored to his desires. The vast majority of the money going into the American health care system has been spent according to the interests and needs of the medical school-trained allopathic physician. Because we accept the doctor's authority without hesitation, because we've never known it to be any other way, we are afraid to challenge the captain of the ship even though we also believe the good ship "U.S.S. Allopathic Medicine" is getting too big and too expensive. We have begun to develop the courage to say we are not going to keep paying for a bigger pie, but we haven't yet thought of changing the ingredients because we implicitly assume only the doctor knows the recipe.

As a consequence of our unquestioning acceptance of the captain's superior and unequaled powers, all other aspects of health care—public health policy, preventive care, alternative (non-allopathic) forms of treatment, and the development of allied health care disciplines—have been relegated to positions of inferior importance. The result is, as *Star Trek's* Mr. (not Dr.) Spock would say, "Quite logical: Our system is defined by allopathic doctors because they have not told us that it can be any other way."

Further, while American medicine might be the best at repairing the human body, it is among the worst of the advanced industrialized nations in keeping its population healthy. Why? Because reducing or eliminating the need to see a doctor is not what the allopathic physician is traditionally paid or trained to do. Primary care physicians, particularly family practitioners, deserve recognition for beginning to integrate meaningful preventive and holistic concepts into their clinical model, but they constitute such a small portion of all doctors that the general point still stands. The vast majority of our doctors practice specialties, not primary care. As we'll see in the concluding chapter of this book, public policy to promote primary care is one of the keys to better health care in the United States. We absolutely must reverse the ratio of primary care providers to medical specialists—something that cannot be done in my lifetime (I'm the same age as President Clinton) unless we allow qualified non-physician providers to have the same level of autonomy enjoyed by physicians.

The "captain of the ship" doctrine is the most far-reaching and enduring result of the Flexner era reforms. By giving the physician sole authority over all other health care providers, it has allowed him to shape twentieth century American health care according to his own desires. Most importantly, it has eliminated all competitors who have a different view of human health, thereby giving the doctor *carte blanche* power to perpetuate the modern medical monopoly.

Authority vs. Professionalism

Being captain of the ship is something very different from being professional. For example, university professors are professionals, but they do not have the authority to prevent outsiders from teaching or researching within their fields. Certified public accountants are at the top of the professional hierarchy of financial scorekeepers, but they cannot prevent public accountants and bookkeepers from preparing our taxes. Architects are the professionals associated with the design of buildings, but they cannot prevent engineers or contractors from making a house. Likewise, attorneys have special roles in the judicial system, but they cannot prevent a real estate agent or consultant from negotiating a contract or resolving a dispute outside the courts.

Physicians are, in effect, the only learned professionals who have managed to place themselves at the top of a hierarchy of other professionals within the same field while controlling the practice of those other professionals (see sidebar: "The Physician's Historical Bill of Rights"). There are, however, a few notable exceptions to this rule of medicine. Dentists, optometrists, podiatrists, and chiropractors have managed to maintain autonomy within limited scopes of practice. In some states, nurse practitioners, nurse midwives, physicians' assistants, and acupuncturists may diagnose and treat on a limited basis, but they are almost always tied to some form of forced relationship with a physician.

The Physician's Historical Bill of Rights

As captain of the ship, the physician has retained ultimate and sole authority over the:

1. *Diagnosis and treatment of illness and injury*

2. *Authorization of all hospital admissions*

3. *Prescription of medicines*

4. *Performance of all surgeries*

With few exceptions, appropriately trained nonphysicians are only allowed to perform these functions under signed orders of a doctor.

Many of the nonphysician health occupations have over the last 20 to 30 years attained recognition as professions in their own right by developing their own clinical models, establishing their own educational requirements, setting their own licensing and certification procedures, gaining their own clinical or scientific bases, developing their own professional ethics, and setting their own standards for quality assurance. The result is now an exceptionally high level of quality in *allied health*—the euphemism assigned to the realm of health care delivered by medical professionals who are not medical doctors. (An even worse generic designation has recently become quite common—*mid-level providers*. I abhor the use of this term to describe the nonphysician providers who have developed the qualifications for independent practice because it still implies an inferiority to the doctor. Would you want to fly on a commercial airliner if the first officer were called a mid-level pilot? The first officer has to be just as skilled in handling the plane as the captain, just as capable of independent action.)

Applying the standards given to most other professions, many of the nonphysician providers should now be allowed to practice independently within their defined areas of clinical specialization. In fact, were we allowed to apply the Flexner-era standards of independent practice today, many nonphysicians would even qualify to be called doctor. However, under the "captain of the ship" doctrine, attainment of professional status has not brought professional independence to many providers who have as much training and skill as doctors in defined areas of clinical practice. They must still act under the direct or general supervision of a doctor because we have not reexamined the foundations of independent practice since the early part of this century. The scientific base of many nonphysician health professions has matured over the past few decades, but the legal foundations of independent practice have not been revised correspondingly. Now is the time for medical law to catch up with medical reality.

The New Armada

Autonomy is something different from professionalism, yet it receives little or no attention from health care policy makers. The issue of professional autonomy—the right to independent practice, to be the captain of one's own ship—can no longer be ignored. Circumstances have changed dramatically in the eight or nine decades since the medical doctor secured authority as the only captain of the only ship. Because of the progress in the abilities and qualifications of non-M.D. health professionals, the United States must now recognize that the "U.S.S. Allopathic Medicine" is not the only ship capable of addressing the problems of human health and that physicians are not the only professionals qualified to set the course.

As we intensify the discussion of various approaches to health care reform, we run the risk of forgetting our purpose. Instead of debating fundamental change of who could deliver health care and who (consumers) would benefit from the expanded supply of substitute providers, we are haggling over little more than different ways to pay for the care that we already have. Even worse, the reform plans being debated in Congress in 1994 implicitly assume that expanding the number of people with health insurance—the quest for universal coverage—is somehow consistent with reducing expenditures on health care.

This approach may sound good to a politician, but it sounds absolutely scary to an economist. Do any of these people remember anything they learned in Economics 101? *Passage of a Clinton-style health reform package would quickly create the classic conditions for inflation: too much money chasing after too few goods.* Of course, most of the health reform plans include mechanisms for price controls, which lead to rationing, which means people get less health care, which is what we set out to avoid in the first place. (No wonder someone once said that the principal cause of problems is solutions!)

This book is an attempt to remind us of a different and economically sensible path to expanding access to affordable health care. While there may never be a permanent solution—solutions will certainly change from generation to generation, and from one medical advancement to another—the quickest, easiest answer to our concurrent problems of limited access and exorbitant cost is already with us. Now is the time to redefine the "captain of the ship" doctrine by launching new ships with nonphysician captains who today meet those very same standards that physicians advanced to create their own monopoly nearly a century ago—captains and ships who will make care affordable and accessible to more people without creating the need for higher taxes or more bureaucracy.

Chapter Five

The Seven Foundations of Professional Autonomy

Abraham Flexner's 1910 report for the Carnegie Foundation did more than expose the wide variations in quality (or lack of it) among the many commercial and educational institutions that trained doctors. The study and related reforms in the medical school curriculum also narrowed the definition of medicine to the science-based, disease-oriented approach of the allopaths. The fallout from Flexner's report, coupled with other changes pushed by the American Medical Association, effectively defined medicine as the sole domain of the scientifically trained physician.

These reforms also helped define the criteria that allopathic doctors used to set themselves up as "captain of the ship" with ultimate authority over all other providers of health care. Though these criteria did not emerge all at once, I have isolated seven criteria as the foundations for independent medical practice—the explicit and implicit arguments physicians historically have used to defend their position as the one and only captain of the one and only ship. This chapter examines these seven foundations of independent practice and shows that doctors are no longer the only health professionals who can meet them.

The foundations of independent practice will continue to evolve in definition and in application. Independent health professionals, both physicians and nonphysicians, could fall short of expectations as the basic requirements of independent practice are modified by advances in knowledge or changes in public expectations. In other words, meeting the requirements of independent practice once should not mean that they are met forever, just as graduating from medical school should not mean that a doctor is forever qualified to practice medicine—which, sadly, has been the case for most of the twentieth century. In recognition of the fact that some doctors become incompetent because they do not keep up with changes in medical practice, some states have recently begun to recertify physicians on a periodic basis. Regular recertification of individual health professionals by state licensing boards makes sense.

Occasional review of individual health professions by state legislatures would be an equally wise move, and now—a period of intense national interest in health care reform—is an ideal time to get started. All independent health professions should be held accountable to these seven foundations of independent practice in exchange for extending to the profession's qualified practitioners the right to diagnose and treat patients on their own, without being held accountable to the captain of another ship.

1. Advanced Education: The Base of Professional Authority

Perhaps the strongest justification for the allopathic medical doctor's ultimate authority came from his extensive education. Because he spent more years in university-based scientific training than any other type of doctor, he presumably knew more than the others and, therefore, possessed the general knowledge to supervise everyone else. This assumption merits reexamination as part of today's needed reforms.

As we have pointed out, at the turn-of-the-century health care was available from a variety of independent practitioners—some academically trained, some not. Many doctors learned by informal apprenticeship, but even the physicians who attended "medical school" were greeted by a tremendous variation in the quality and length of the curriculum. While a handful of excellent, university-affiliated schools eventually provided the model for our current system of four years of medical education, there were at the same time many "diploma mills" where a doctor's training could be completed in a matter of months. Few schools for would-be doctors required any college education for admission, and most lacked basic laboratory facilities. On the whole, Abraham Flexner concluded, medical education varied from generally inadequate to "utterly wretched." There were a few good examples—Harvard, the University of Pennsylvania, and particularly Johns Hopkins—which offered students adequate facilities and required four years of post-baccalaureate, college-level education for an M.D. degree, including some practical training (see sidebar: "What's in a Title?").

The current four-year requirement for medical study is based on the curriculum adopted in 1892 by the medical school at Johns Hopkins University, which Abraham Flexner placed at the top of his rankings of American medical schools. At the time, Flexner deemed four years an adequate period to master the art and science of medicine. Four years probably was adequate, given the medical knowledge of the day. Of course, at the same time students could enter commercial medical schools with little or no college education, and once they graduated they were free to "hang out a shingle." Johns Hopkins, on the other hand, required some college preparation before admission to its medical school.

In the 1990s, the minimum training for a physician has been expanded to somewhere between six and eight years of post-secondary education, including two to four years of undergraduate education—but not necessarily a bachelor's degree—and four years of medical school. Most doctors today also receive specialty training in medical residencies lasting from three to five years. However, residency training is not a requirement of becoming a captain of the ship; only the M.D. degree and state licensure are required for entry into independent practice. Today, some students even enter medical school with graduate degrees in a variety of fields. Three reasons account for this increase in a typical doctor's years of training.

- First, once the medical education reform movement began, the medical schools with minimum admissions standards went out of business. Those schools with more stringent admissions standards could afford to raise them even higher due to the increased competition for fewer student slots. Some college- or university-level education—even a bachelor's degree—became common as students began to compete with one another for a smaller number of medical school openings.

- Second, the overall knowledge of medicine began to expand dramatically. Instead of expanding the curriculum or raising requirements for graduation, medical schools left the majority of specialty training to take place later as hospital-based residencies and internships—an institutionalization of the old apprenticeship system.

- The third reason for inflation in medical training was money. By the early 1960s, doctors' salaries and social status had risen to unprecedented levels. Specialization was the key to the future. Doctors, having gained the unchallenged power to set their own fees, realized the more technical the procedure they could perform, the more money they could ask for it.

The increase in training meant an increase in the cost of physicians' services, but the payers—primarily insurance companies—weren't expressing any concerns. Insurance companies found that they could easily cover their increased costs by passing the bill on to America's employers, who in turn could absorb increased insurance costs as untaxed "benefits" for their employees. When Medicare and Medicaid arrived in 1965, the federal government essentially committed itself to pick up the slack in the system—that is, cover the costs of care for the elderly and poor who were least likely to have insurance. The money was there to pay doctors for new skills created by extended training and specialization; all they had to do was ask for it.

Adding an internship and residency to a physician's training was as economically desirable as it was clinically necessary. Specialization was beginning to net doctors noticeably increased financial returns. Residencies and internships—despite their long hours, sleep deprivation, and low pay—were rightly seen as an investment leading to even better income.

What's in a Title?

To this day, the M.D. is technically an undergraduate college degree, and a high school diploma is the only degree requirement for acceptance into medical school. The current expectation that students who enter medical school must have an undergraduate degree is a result of the increasing competition to enter medical school once the profession gained its monopoly powers. Contrary to popular belief, some students who enter medical school even now have not attained a bachelor's degree.

In some ways, medical school is a cross between a university and a technical school: the first two years focus on the academic study of medicine, the last two on practical, "hands-on" experience. From the traditional academic point of view, recipients of the medical degree should not be called "doctor" because they have not received the scholarly equivalent of a Ph.D. Indeed, in most other countries in the world where medical students complete a four-year curriculum equivalent to the offering of a medical school in the United States, the graduate doctor is still called "Mister." The American doctor's success in gaining a distinguished social title is yet another sign of the extraordinary power that physicians have gained in this country.

Although specialization required increased education, the core curriculum in medical school remained essentially unchanged. With competition for admission causing more and more applicants to get an undergraduate degree before entering medical school, medical students often found themselves taking the same courses they had in college (some of which, like organic chemistry, were prerequisites for admission!). Furthermore, they were still required to take the four-year core curriculum even if they had already decided to pursue a specialty that required only a portion of the core curriculum's content. Thus, a student intending to become an ophthalmologist would still spend 10 weeks learning how to deliver a baby, another 10 weeks learning how to set bones, and yet a third, fourth or fifth 10-week block similarly immersed in another medical study just as distant from his chosen specialty. (This broad approach is not necessarily bad in the context of multidisciplinary education; many of us are enriched professionally and personally by studying a variety of subjects that are not directly related to our day-to-day activities. However, given the very high cost of medical education, we should perhaps be asking if the extra exposure is worth the extra cost. After 20 years of involvement in medical education, I think some cost-benefit analysis of the curriculum is in order.)

Medicine as practiced in the late twentieth century is vastly different from the way it was practiced back when being a doctor meant being a generalist. Today, the opposite is true. The vast majority of today's doctors become specialists. But the medical school curriculum does not reflect that shift. Undergraduate medical students must still complete four years of training that were designed for a career—general medicine—that very few of them will follow. This turn of events does not challenge advanced education as a requirement for independent practice. It does show that the four years of medical school is not a gold standard for anything in particular.

As I have previously mentioned, a few independent health care professions were able to escape the M.D. umbrella created by the medical reforms of the early 1900s. Podiatry and dentistry are proof that carefully defined areas of independent practice can exist *separately* from general medicine rather than as *an extended branch of* general medicine operating only under doctors' orders. These independent medical specialties offer a rational and efficient alternative to the traditional medical education.

Specialization begins the day the student enters the school of dentistry or podiatry. All training relates directly to clinical practice; no time is spent learning general medical skills (e.g., delivering a baby, casting a broken arm) that will never be done again. Then, after four years of carefully focused training, graduates are perfectly capable of competent practice limited to the mouth or foot, respectively. Although a bachelor's degree is generally required for students entering podiatry or dental schools, an extensive residency afterwards is not necessary because the four-year curriculum was designed for specialization. Further training is necessary only if a graduate of these programs wishes to become a subspecialist, such as a dentist choosing to go into orthodontics.

Practicing dentists and podiatrists provide a very good—but regrettably rare—example of the viability of competent, competitive clinical practice without the oversight of a physician. Both, for example, offer some services that are also provided by orthopedic surgeons who spend more than twice as much time in medical training—time that includes a lot of courses not even remotely related to bones and ligaments in the mouth or foot. The unquestioned existence of dentistry and podiatry as independent professions should give us confidence to engage in new thinking about the requirements for becoming a captain of a ship. The plain fact is that four years of medical school is no longer a meaningful requirement for independent practice. It is instead a tradition that unjustifiably excludes all but a handful of other health care professionals from being captains of their own ships.

This conclusion does not mean that the turn-of-the-century reformers had the wrong idea. At that time, minimum educational standards needed to be set for independent practice. The same is certainly true today. But the issue is setting currently defensible standards, not blindly accepting the century-old medical school curriculum as the minimum standard for all time. Having gone to medical school was once a sound criterion, but it is no longer a justification for the monopoly power to exclude other qualified professionals from independent practice.

Any qualified health profession should be allowed within the scope of law to define and defend the minimum education needed to prepare a qualified student for entry into independent practice. These minimum educational requirements should include guidelines for the appropriate mix of classroom and clinical training from the general university, the specialty school, and the residency program. Admittedly, the minimums will vary by profession in order to reflect differences among the various scopes of clinical practice and underlying knowledge. For example, a surgeon may need nine years of professional training, while an independent physical therapist might need only five. Similarly, a basic primary care provider, such as a nurse practitioner, hardly needs eight or nine years of training to check for earaches and sore throats or to suture uncomplicated lacerations.

Years of education are not the only determinants of clinical competence. For example, psychiatrists have completed four years of medical school but are generally unqualified to deal with critical life-and-death emergency situations involving trauma or physical illness. On the other hand, paramedics with less than a year of training can be highly skilled at saving lives. And orthopedic surgeons, who are the only professionals currently qualified to perform knee surgery, do not possess the physical therapist's superb skills in getting a limb, a joint, or a back working again after a debilitating injury.

The Flexner era reforms of medical education were not uniformly embraced by the profession. Some physicians warned against making medicine overly scientific at the expense of a broader, more humanistic approach. Others objected to requiring a rigorous general education for all physicians prior to selecting a special area of concentration. Still others foresaw the coming disappearance of those schools that could not fit in with the more elitist university-type education, including medical colleges catering to blacks, women, and poor students. In the end, these predictions came true, and the medical profession grew comfortably into its role as a group of white, upper-class men armed with the latest scientific advancements, riding into battle against injury and disease. Something important was lost in the process.

In short, while the turn-of-the-century reforms in medical education insured adequate basic training for the generalist physician, they have by the end of the century become expensive, wasteful, and exclusionary. We will see in subsequent chapters that there are now a number of other health professions with an advanced educational base. While that base may not be as broad as that of the pre-specialization doctor, it is more than ample to qualify those providers for independent practice in their respective fields of expertise.

2. Ongoing Certification

The education of a health care provider does not stop with a degree. Educational competency in any health profession is made up of two components: educational base and ongoing training. The two are distinguished from one another because they imply very different skills. Getting a degree provides a future health care practitioner with the scientific and clinical base to be a lifelong learner. Continuing education, on the other hand, indicates the practitioner is keeping up with all the various scientific and methodological advances in a given field or is additionally choosing to expand upon his or her educational base to pick up new health care skills.

Given today's fast-paced revolution in the foundations of clinical practice, all health professionals must devote many hours each week to keeping up with all the changes in medical science and technology. I believe that the half-life of what a future physician learns in medical school today is somewhere between two and three years. (My physician friends have their own half-life estimates in the same general range.) In other words, half the knowledge a medical student picks up during the course of his formal studies is replaced by new knowledge in three years or less. Some of it becomes outdated, the rest is simply inapplicable.

This decay of medical school knowledge continues throughout the physician's career, so that within five to 10 years the physician needs to develop a knowledge base that is almost completely new and different from what he learned in medical school. A good physician will constantly replace this old knowledge with what he learns through experience and continuing educational programs. But experience or ongoing training alone are not enough to insure clinical competency. Periodic recertification is also a desirable requirement for renewal of the right to be captain of a ship.

Until the latter part of the nineteenth century, most doctors in the United States were apprenticeship-trained; they did not receive a formal medical education in a school or university as we know it today. This gradually changed as medical training became more a degree than an apprenticeship. However, most of these schools were not affiliated with a university. They were more like trade schools, and some began graduating students into practice after a very short academic period with little or no "hands-on" training. By the beginning of the twentieth century, book learning had been added to clinical learning in most of America's medical schools.

Academic training and experience still go hand-in-hand. A physician whose practice is based solely on what he learned in medical school is quite likely a danger to patients. A doctor who does not continue to educate himself in the rapidly unfolding advances in medical science—new technologies, drugs, diagnostic procedures, surgical methods, even diseases—should not continue to practice even though he went to medical school. Fortunately, most states require physicians to take continuing medical education (CME) courses for relicensure.

Certain professional societies, such as the American Academy of Family Practice or the American College of Emergency Physicians, additionally require a program of ongoing education and certification for physicians to retain membership. There is no consistent national standard, however, across the United States. Depending on where he or she sets up practice, a physician can theoretically graduate from medical school, enter practice ("hang out a shingle," in the old vernacular) and pursue no other course of study throughout his or her lifetime. In other words, earning the M.D. degree is not by itself justification for a permanent right to independent practice, and doctors use a meaningless argument when trying to deny the privilege to nonphysician providers because they haven't been to medical school.

As noted in the previous section, periodic certification for physicians is becoming more common; it is also becoming more rigorous. Most specialty societies require not only medical school training, but a completed residency and a certain number of years of supervised patient care. Physicians must also recertify their skills every few years in most medical specialties by taking an examination to demonstrate up-to-date competency. Until just recently, doctors only had to prove they did not have any problems in their practice and that they had taken a specified number of hours of CME. More and more, medical boards are even requiring physicians to take written examinations every few years for recertification, a procedure I wholeheartedly endorse as one of the absolute requirements of independent practice for any health profession.

However, my endorsement of the physicians' good example in promoting recertification does not mean that physicians should also control the recertification of independent nonphysician providers with advanced practice skills. Allied health personnel are generally under the rigorous control of state boards, which are often controlled by physicians. Ironically, allied health professionals can find themselves subject to more rigorous certification procedures than the physicians who employ, control, and monitor them. Qualified nonphysician providers should be required to follow the physicians' good example of ongoing recertification on their own, without physician control.

If this nation is going to end the doctors' monopoly over its health care delivery system—as it must if we are to lower costs by ensuring competitive choice—the states need to establish consistent certification and recertification standards for all independent health care providers. No one profession should be able to exclude qualified competitors from the market by controlling the certification process. In fact, certification standards could—and perhaps should—cross professional boundaries. If a nurse midwife must periodically demonstrate up-to-date competence in certain obstetrical procedures, so should a family practice doctor who wishes to handle comparable deliveries. While medical education and licensing set the groundwork for the independent practice of medicine, certification of specific competence can guarantee a consistently high level of practice across the professions and assure ongoing learning throughout a medical career. Certification should be a strict requirement for the right to independent practice, but physicians should not control the certification process of other autonomous health professions. Everyone ought to play by the same rules, so the challenge is to develop an acceptable general model of certification—not to encompass the other health professions within the doctors' model.

3. Scientific Base

Adherence to scientific principles is one of the key criteria that allopathic physicians used so effectively to build their educational, clinical, and economic monopoly. At the allopaths' insistence, clinical paradigms not based on scientific methods were eliminated by state medical practice acts in the early decades of the twentieth century. (Just to be perfectly clear, I think this was the right and good thing to do. I teach research and scientific method at a medical school, and I am a strong defender of the scientific base of clinical practice.) Thanks to the work of Pasteur and other scientists in the last half of the nineteenth century, this rejection of unscientific clinical models came at a period when—perhaps for the first time in human history—medicine could effect a cure and begin to explain why the cure worked.

Many of scientific medicine's competitors during the turn-of-the-century era of medical reform deserved to be put out of business because their approaches were demonstrably ineffective or did more harm than good. Many nonphysician providers lacked any formal scientific training whatsoever. Furthermore, purveyors of so-called patent medicines hawked their goods freely and did not have to prove the effectiveness or safety of their proprietary preparations.

Scientific research has substantially reduced this problem. Even though physicians have received the lion's share of research funding from government and private sources, the nonphysician health professionals have benefited from the scientific base that allopathic medicine has provided. Furthermore, nonphysician providers have developed their own research bases, with scholarly articles published in their own refereed journals (see sidebar: "How Do We Know If It's Scientific?").

A strong scientific base is not only important in determining the legitimacy of an intervention, but also in identifying ineffective or even harmful treatments. Doctors would like us to believe that we always benefit from their care, but medical intervention is not always helpful. Indeed, much care is unnecessary because the normal human body has remarkable curative powers of its own. A significant portion of the ills that cause a person to see a doctor are self-limiting; they will resolve in due course with or without medical intervention. (Doctors have an old saying that they can help a patient get rid of the common cold in just seven days if the patient does everything the doctor orders. On the other hand, a sufferer who does nothing for the cold can usually expect it to last for a whole week.) Until a cure can be found for the common cold, for instance, there is no reason to seek professional help, except to see if something else is wrong if the symptoms persist for an unreasonably long time.

How Do We Know If It's Scientific?

The primary measure of a scientific base is the existence of a literature published in rigorously refereed journals that enforce adherence to accepted principles of scientific research and statistical analysis. This published literature is based on random and controlled clinical trials that demonstrate whether any observed difference associated with treatment is or is not likely caused by a specific medical treatment—the experimental effect.

The scientific integrity of medicine's published literature has been far from perfect in the past, but it is getting better. Recent improvements may stem from American science's efforts to police itself in response to growing charges of fraud and sloppiness in medical research. Several respected journals have recently strengthened the rigor of their editorial policies, making them models for the publications of other health professions. An important criterion of independent practice is met by any health profession that can produce scientific literature comparable to most studies currently found in the New England Journal of Medicine, *the* Journal of the American Medical Association, *or* Science.

Unfortunately, medical care itself can cause harm, giving the patient a problem that he or she did not have when first going to the physician for treatment. Indeed, doctor-induced illness is sufficiently common to have merited a formal name: *iatrogenic* disease. Not much of this is due to physician negligence. In fact, the vast majority of iatrogenic disease has occurred as a result of scientific ignorance. Medical history is littered with accepted treatments that have subsequently been found to be questionable or even do more harm than good. Drugs that were once in favor and easily available (e.g., cocaine and DES) have created problems far worse than those they were reputed to cure. Another tragic example of such error is thalidomide, which caused thousands of birth defects in the early 1960s. Many medicines on the market today may not have any physical effect on the illnesses or symptoms they purport to alleviate. What they are doing otherwise to the body is often unknown. Surgery has also been overused. Tonsillectomies, hysterectomies, cesarean sections, and heart bypass operations have all become common—and all are now being challenged as unnecessary in a large number of cases. English doctors, for example, perform far fewer open heart surgeries than their American counterparts, and the French choose fewer radical mastectomies for breast cancer, preferring lumpectomies instead. The English and the French are no less healthy even though they get much less surgery.

In other words, medical science is not perfect. However, it has matured considerably during this century, and the scientific base of modern medicine has grown along with it. American medicine today follows consistent scientific practices that can serve as a generally acceptable model for judging the practices of *all* health professions that want the right to independent practice (see sidebar: "The French Connection"). The scientific deficiencies of the medical doctor's turn-of-the-century competitors do not justify a permanent injunction against today's nonphysician providers who have built their own scientifically defensible foundations. Just because allopathic medicine was the first profession to comply with the principle of having a scientific base as a prerequisite for independent practice, it does not qualify doctors to hold a permanent monopoly over health care. *If other health providers are willing to play by the same scientific rules, they ought to be allowed to get on the same playing field.*

The French Connection

I grew to accept the medical monopoly at an early age. There were several physicians in my family, and I always had doctors for any medical care I needed. I just assumed that doctors were the people you went to when you had a health problem and that there was only one kind of doctor—the kind that went to medical school.

One night as a student living in France in 1968, I greatly overindulged in champagne and chocolate. The next morning, I thought I was going to die. It was more than a hangover; it was "whole body pain." I was barely able to function.

I asked the French lady in whose home I was staying to please call a doctor. "What kind of a doctor would you like?" she asked.

"A doctor," I said. I spoke French well, so I knew I wasn't miscommunicating. "You know, a doctor."

"Fine," she repeated, "but I need to know what kind of doctor you'd like."

Suddenly, it occurred to me in my miserable state that we were experiencing a cultural problem here. Many different kinds of doctors are allowed to practice medicine in France. France never had a Flexner Report, nor did it go through the medical reforms that gave the sole medical franchise to the scientifically trained M.D. in the United States. In France in 1968, various kinds of doctors that had been drummed out of business in the United States were still in business. Naturopaths, homeopaths, faith healers, and herbalists all were available to me, and all were reimbursed by the national health plan.

This was the first time in my life that I had ever realized there could be more than one approach to medicine and that someone other than a medical school graduate might be accepted in a civilized country. Ultimately I chose a traditional allopathic doctor to help me through my "illness," but the sudden awareness that I had this choice was one of those rare moments in life when I really felt the unforgettable jolt of a paradigm being shifted. It might even be identified as the moment when this book began to take shape.

Because medicine is not absolute, today's folk remedy or experimental treatment may be tomorrow's medical science. Conversely, today's accepted therapy may be relegated to the annals of medical history as a laughable instance of ignorance or tragic medical blundering. While I acknowledge the potential value of some nontraditional therapies, I do not propose to relax the scientific foundations of independent clinical practice. *Science may not solve all problems of human health, but efforts to provide doctors with much-needed competition will almost surely fail if independent practitioners are not held to the same scientific standards as physicians.*

In the absence of something better than science, we should remember the Hippocratic Oath's charge to the healer, "Above all, do no harm." In answering to this dictum, all health care personnel—be they physician or otherwise—are equally responsible. Scientific method is the best tool we have to judge our performance according to this standard. It has served allopathic medicine well, but it is a tool that can and must be used by all independent health professionals.

4. Coherent Clinical Model

Modern, mainstream medicine is not much more than one hundred years old. Until Louis Pasteur discovered the bacterial cause of disease in the 1860s, doctors had weak scientific foundations for understanding disease and knowing how to treat it. The understanding of disease that existed before Pasteur was based on subjective experience rather than objective understanding. For hundreds of years prior to Pasteur's discovery, doctors diagnosed by sensory perception and treated by various methods that seem barbaric by today's standards because they did not know any better. For example, smelling and tasting a patient's urine was a key diagnostic method, and bloodletting with leeches was a principal "cure."

The medical revolution represented by Pasteur's discoveries did not cause the immediate disappearance of non-allopathic approaches to medicine. Other models of human health continued to exist, and although they were based more on theory than fact, each did embody an internally consistent and independent set of clinical concepts. Schools of clinical practice were categorized according to the distinctly different conceptual foundations of their approach.[1] For example, following the ancient saying that like things are cured by like things, the school of homeopathy relied on small doses of antagonist agents—poisonous in larger doses—to induce reactions that would presumably cure a disease. The school of humoralism (from the Latin word, *umere*, "to be moist") relied on analysis of the body's secretions for clues to the cause of illness, and herbalism sought cure through the ingestion of dried plants believed to have specific medicinal properties. Each of these schools follows a different model in approaching the same disease.

Chiropractic, established in 1895, explained illness as a function of a misaligned nervous system and pursued cure through a realignment of the spine. Osteopathy began about the same time and also purported that disease was a function of misalignment, though of the various parts of the body in addition to the spinal column. Its cure called for manipulation of the joints. In addition to sharing spinal manipulation as part of their respective clinical models, osteopaths and chiropractors also share a strong focus on preventive medicine, a clinical concept that the allopathic-dominated medical monopoly has for the most part chosen to ignore. In spite of allopaths' strenuous objections, osteopathic and chiropractic models of illness and cure have survived as alternatives to the allopathic monopoly, though on relatively smaller scales.

Originally, like the allopathic medical schools of the day, chiropractic and osteopathic colleges offered a course of study that competed with the standard undergraduate education. Today, both require undergraduate study as an admission requirement, and both offer a standardized curriculum in their respective four-year colleges. However, osteopaths are accorded by state medical practice acts all the same privileges as allopaths, including access to hospitals and the right to prescribe drugs. Most osteopaths also pursue a residency (often an allopathic residency) following medical school and take the same national examinations as allopathic doctors. Osteopaths are increasingly accepted by allopaths. Chiropractors, on the other hand, cannot prescribe

---

1. Specific definitions are taken from William S. Haubrich's *Medical Meanings: A Glossary of Word Origins* (San Diego: Harcourt Brace Jovanovich, 1984) and *Mosby's Medical and Nursing Dictionary*, 2nd edition (St. Louis: C.V. Mosby Company, 1986).

drugs in most states and have only recently gained the right to some hospital privileges. To allopaths, the chiropractic model of medical care is viewed as unscientific.

Allopathy and osteopathy are not the only internally consistent clinical models for approaching the problems of human health. Other defensible paradigms exist within the allied health professions—nonphysician models that now deserve a right to compete independently in the medical marketplace. In other words, a doctor should not have the right to control access to the practitioners of other clinical models when those models are scientifically defensible and internally consistent in ways that permit rational choice by informed consumers.

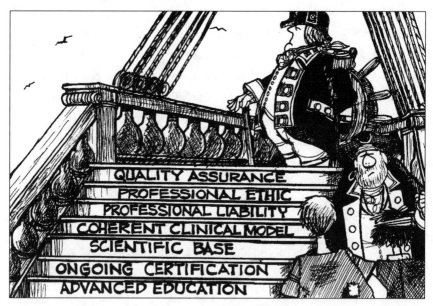

Opening the medical marketplace to competing clinical models—including physical therapy, audiology, respiratory therapy, and nursing (nurse practitioners and nurse midwives)—can give consumers an added dimension of choice that has been missing in the United States since allopathic medicine secured its monopoly in the early decades of this century. The AMA and other bulwarks of organized medicine have carefully maintained an illusion of competition by defending the patient's right to choose a doctor, but they have deprived the nation of a richer form and higher order of competition—the right to choose among independent practitioners of different clinical models.

5. Professional Liability

Together, a scientific base and a coherent clinical model can provide specific criteria for a defensible form of practice. The scientific base divides proven from unproven (or disproven) approaches within the clinical model. A professional who steps outside the boundaries of competence within his or her defined clinical model is guilty of negligent practice and, consistent with our heritage of tort law, deserves punishment corresponding with the extent of the deviation and the resulting harm.

As "captains of the ship," physicians have unhesitatingly accepted liability not only for their own actions, but for those of their crew as well. (Acceptance, however, is different from enforcement—the subject of the seventh criterion for independent practice, "Quality Assurance.") Doctors' professional associations do not intervene in the judicial process in defense of a doctor who has obviously practiced negligently, nor do they have a record of promoting legislation that would weaken consumers' fair recourse against a doctor guilty of malpractice. Similarly, doctors do not commonly attempt to evade responsibility when a subordinate commits an error that harms a patient. To its enduring credit, organized medicine does not have a "buyer beware" skeleton in its closet, as is the case in the history of most other monopolies in the American economy.

Just as physicians have accepted professional liability, so must other health care providers who choose to practice independently. The rules of the game of professional liability must be applied to *all* independent practitioners hanging out their shingles. None of the qualified nonphysician providers should be exempt from the same legal concepts and mechanisms of professional liability that apply to the practice of medicine. Of course, the movement for malpractice reform (easily the subject of another book) may ultimately produce improvements in the way we deal with doctors' negligence, but any future changes in medical malpractice should be equally applicable to the captains of other ships. In other words, creating some competition for doctors does not create any special malpractice issues as long as the newly independent practitioners are clearly held accountable to the same legal standards.

Although I do not believe that qualified nonphysician providers should receive any special treatment with respect to professional liability, I do favor the exploration of alternatives to traditional methods for enforcing it. For example, the transfer of liability from the practitioner to the institution that employs doctors and other independent providers is perhaps a viable option. Institutional liability—also called enterprise liability—might promote quality control among the provider organizations or professional societies because then they would be ultimately responsible for the actions of their employees or members. Such a system would limit costs created by multiple-tier lawsuits where, for example, both the physician and the hospital are sued. The idea merits further study.

The launching of new ships captained by qualified nonphysician professionals may initially give the appearance of creating liability problems because many of the newly independent providers will need to refer their patients to a physician for services that are not within their scope of practice. For example, a nurse midwife who is fully qualified to handle a normal delivery all by herself may need to refer to an obstetrician an expectant mother who during the course of prenatal care is discovered to be a high-risk patient. Or a physical therapist who is fully qualified to diagnose and treat a sprained ankle may discover an unrelated bone defect that requires the attention of an orthopedic surgeon. Failure to refer the patient to the appropriate physician would constitute negligent practice.

Neither of these examples is any different from the situation occurring in the office of a physician in general or family practice. Any doctor engages in negligent practice when he attempts to diagnose or treat a condition outside his scope of practice. Existing law governing referrals, with appropriate language to cover the addition of nonphysician providers, should suffice to regulate this situation adequately. New law is not needed, and the issue of legal responsibility for referral should not be used to prevent patients from having direct access to qualified independent practitioners with carefully defined scopes of practice. Many doctors have to refer their patients to specialists; I see no reason why qualified nonphysician providers cannot be trusted to do the same.

The process of extending full liability to qualified nonphysician providers would also be a good occasion for bringing the whole tort system back to a proper concept of negligent practice. Health professionals should only be found guilty of malpractice when they fail to do the right thing, i.e., when they do not adhere to accepted standards of practice. Due to the vagaries of the human condition, a poor outcome is not necessarily proof that a doctor did anything wrong. All independent health practitioners should be liable for the appropriateness of their actions, not for the result of their care.

Scientific research should be constantly updating the standards of care against which all independent practitioners—including physicians—are judged. In this regard, the accelerating development of clinical practice guidelines supports expanding the number of qualified independent health professionals. A considerable amount of research is now directed at identifying the most cost-effective of alternative approaches to treating a particular illness, allowing the development of formal principles to guide clinicians in their diagnosis and treatment. Insurance reimbursement is being tied to adherence to accepted guidelines.

For example, a clinical practice guideline for a specific condition might indicate that a course of drugs should be tried for two weeks as an alternative to immediate surgery because the drug usually works and costs a whole lot less than the surgery. The surgery would be approved for reimbursement only after the drug therapy has failed, unless the doctor can first show that the patient is a special case falling outside the guideline. Much of what physicians have called the "art" of medical practice is now becoming part of the "science," and doctors have no unique claim to science. Further, nonphysician providers have been following practice guidelines—called doctors' orders—for years; they should be at least as qualified as doctors in working with this growing foundation of clinical practice.

6. Professional Ethic

The ethics of a profession are the shared guidelines—both written and unwritten—that define the commonly accepted conduct of a professional practice. Until the mid-1970s, medicine's code of ethics dealt almost entirely with how doctors should relate to one another rather than how they should deal with patients. The ethics of the doctor-patient relationship were governed by custom arising out of the Hippocratic Oath, which had been regularly reinterpreted to fit the prevailing thought of the medical era. The Oath's clear statement "Above all, do no harm," quite clearly has been amended by another, stronger doctrine reflective of medicine's newfound power over nature and the legal system's expanded expectations: "Above all, do whatever possible to keep the patient alive [my phrasing]."

The professional ethic of American medicine exists on several levels. The first is practitioner to patient. Here, despite the historical lack of written guidelines, the vast number of doctors have achieved high marks. However, more and more care is moving from a doctor-patient relationship to an institution-patient relationship, with more of the one-on-one care relegated to nurses and other allied health personnel. Of course, some physicians have used their professional position either to practice bad medicine or to take advantage of their patients, a problem exacerbated by the reluctance of physicians to police their own colleagues. (Indeed, letters of recommendation for a physician who is looking for a new position can be motivated by a desire to get rid of an undesirable colleague.)

Another level of professional ethic is the physician's responsibility to society, and here the medical monopoly has let us down. Doctors have enjoyed an enormous increase in income and social prestige at a time when access to medical care has sadly become a function of the patient's ability to pay. As Jacques Barzun said about physicians (and to a lesser extent about teachers and lawyers), "The modern professions have enjoyed their monopoly for so long that they have forgotten that it is a privilege given in exchange for a public benefit."[2] Too many physicians have become detached from the original mission of healer and caregiver and are now using the system as a means toward a well-funded lifestyle.

"What every profession should bear in mind," Barzun warned, "is the distinction between a profession and a function. The function may well be eternal; but the profession, which is the cluster of practices and relationships arising from the function at a given time and place, can be destroyed—or can destroy itself—very rapidly." While it is foolhardy to predict the end of doctors—there

---

2. From "The Professions under Siege," originally published in *Harper's*, October 1978.

will always be a need for highly trained medical specialists—the *medical pro-fession* needs to return to its ethical heritage of public service. The same must be expected of all other health professionals who claim the right to independent practice.

At no point does the Hippocratic Oath say, "I bequeath this charge only to people who go to medical school in the twentieth century." There are other well-educated and highly experienced health care professionals waiting for an opportunity to practice what they have been trained to do on their own. Their professional ethics are just as important as those of the physician. The non-physician providers must also prove themselves responsible not only to the individual patient, but to the society as a whole. Ethically, there is no reason to deny patients access to legitimate nonphysician providers simply because those providers have not graduated from medical school, as long as they are willing to adhere to the same ethical standards that are the proud heritage—if not always the current practice—of America's physicians.

7. Quality Assurance

From the mid-1960s through the 1980s, professional peer review was the standard method for evaluating the quality of care provided by physicians. The meaning of peer review is as simple as it sounds: doctors evaluate other doctors. It operates under the joint assumptions that (1) doctors and only doctors know what is best for patients, and (2) the only person qualified to judge a doctor's work is another doctor. This is similar to allowing, for example, airline pilots to be the only judges of airline pilots, oil tanker captains to be the only judges of oil tanker captains, nuclear waste disposal technicians to be the only judges of nuclear waste disposal technicians, etc.

Peer review among physicians has in the last decade given way to other forms of review because it is imperfect. All too often, it has perpetuated the "good old boy" network at the expense of the patient. When physicians are called upon to evaluate each other's work, they can easily be caught in a conflict of interest. Physicians called upon to review their peers ultimately must decide whether their allegiance lies with the physician or with the patient. The doctor under review is a fellow professional—a member of the fraternity. Often he is a co-worker and quite possibly a personal friend, which raises questions about objectivity. Further, the legal system provides the reviewing doctor with very weak protection against suits from physicians whose care is evaluated negatively. Finally, medicine is not an exact science, and often the difference between the right or wrong decision is hidden within a very large gray area, subject to personal interpretation of peer reviewers.

To their credit, doctors have recently begun to employ new and different methods of physician review. One is using data-based systems. Information is taken from patient records, coded, and analyzed for deviations from the norms. For any diagnosis, pertinent questions can then be answered: Were the correct procedures completed? Were the right tests performed? Were they performed at the right time? Were any unnecessary tests performed? What drugs were prescribed? What did the doctor tell the patient? What was the outcome of the treatment? (Clinical practice guidelines are rapidly emerging as the source of answers to these questions.)

Let's take an example of a patient who enters a hospital with chest pains and who later dies. A preliminary inquiry into the patient's care raises some question as to whether he received appropriate treatment. Under peer review, a group of physicians, who may or may not be experts in cardiopulmonology, looks at the record. They ultimately determine that while some of the steps taken by the attending physician were not customary, there is inconclusive evidence as to whether the physician made a gross error. In a data-based review, an impartial expert can go through that record and determine whether the action taken with the patient followed given protocols and complied with acceptable norms. The gray area may still exist, but at least it is placed into a context outside the realm of the close personal relationships.

Historically, the allopathic physician has had to balance his science as a doctor and his art as a healer. Certainly, healing at the end of the twentieth century is still not a purely scientific endeavor. The modern physician must keep one foot in each of two worlds: the world of scientific evidence and the world of personal experience. Yet peer review judges him on another level altogether—that is, whether or not he conforms to the accepted norms of a peer group. A brilliant doctor can fail in peer review simply because he or she doesn't get along with the group. Data-based review at least holds the doctor accountable to medical science, which is the primary foundation on which he has staked his monopoly over twentieth century medicine. Fortunately, data-based analyses have become common in America's hospitals. In fact, the hospital industry has arguably been the leader in bringing improvements to the realm of quality assurance, but we cannot count on hospitals to manage this function in the long run because more and more medical care is being delivered on an outpatient basis. The reimbursement system is the lowest common denominator for administering quality assessment in the future—but it, too, is an imperfect mechanism because withholding payment is not enough to correct problems.

Quality assurance must be corrective. It must include mechanisms that educate doctors whose practices deviate from the acceptable norm. For example, if the medical literature indicates that patients only benefit from a particular drug under certain circumstances and a patient was administered the drug despite a total absence of these circumstances, then the physician needs to be told in a constructive manner that what he did was outside the norm, and given suggestions for improving future performance.

Quality assurance has probably been the weakest of the seven foundations for doctors' claims of professional superiority. Nevertheless, meaningful assessment with appropriate corrective mechanisms must be accepted by any providers who practice independently. Ironically, nonphysician providers—the nurses, audiologists, physical therapists, pharmacists, etc.—have historically been subject to more scrutiny than the doctors. Because they have always worked *for or under* doctors, they have been automatically subject to review by an outsider, i.e., a physician. Review standards have remained both independent and stringent for nonphysician providers, making it far easier, for example, to fire an incompetent nurse than get rid of an inept doctor.

Regardless of the history of quality assurance as practiced by doctors, the central concept of criteria-based review by an independent authority must be accepted by any health care personnel who want to diagnose and treat patients as independent providers. Commercial airline pilots are as responsible as doctors for the lives of others, and their performance can be evaluated at any time and without warning by an FAA inspector. The same rigorous review by a qualified outsider should be expected of any health professional—including doctors.

Rebuilding from the Ground Up

The foundations for independent medical practice are not what is wrong with the system. In tallying up the scorecard, we see that most doctors meet all seven of these criteria, and the criteria continue to make sense. Physicians have provided a generally strong case for justifying their right to independent practice. However, we all know that some physicians do not meet these criteria. Physicians must no longer be allowed to deprive other qualified providers of the right to independent practice simply because the others are not perfect, i.e., because they are not doctors. Doctors are not perfect, either, but that fact has not kept them from being captain of a ship.

Using these seven foundations of independent practice, we can easily identify some nonphysician providers of medical care who meet the criteria to be captains of their own ships. The qualified nonphysician practitioners of these professions receive an extensive educational background. Their professions have established programs for ongoing certification. They can cite a strong scientific base to support their interventions. They are well-grounded in their unique and coherent clinical models. They are willing to accept professional liability. They have an established professional ethic. And they can make a strong commitment to quality assurance. Today's qualified nonphysicians should not be denied independent practice simply because doctors were the only health professionals who met these expectations when they wrote the rules to eliminate unqualified competitors at the beginning of the twentieth century.

The chapters in the following part of this book examine in detail these nonphysicians qualified for independent practice and show how their competitive entry into the medical marketplace would make health care for Americans both *more accessible* and *less costly* without producing any harmful changes in the quality of care. Better yet, we will see how this competitive approach accomplishes the goals of health care reform without creating the need for tax increases and new bureaucracies.

Chapter Six

New Choices on the Menu: The Independent Nurses

The doctors' monopoly makes American medicine somewhat analogous to broadcast television that offers only network stations—evening programming has very little variety, one sitcom looks exactly like another, and the network news on ABC looks remarkably like the news on CBS and NBC, with all covering the same events with similar sound bites and editorial comments. While some viewers are satisfied with the broadcast television fare that is presented to them day after day, others were becoming so disillusioned that they would rather shut the television off completely and bury their heads in a newspaper or novel.

Well, defectors have been lured back to their television screens by the greater selection of programming made available through cable—an incredibly successful medium due to its ability to respond to a wide variety of tastes. For example, persons craving freedom from editorial bias can replace broadcast news shows with C-SPAN. Others can watch the news at odd hours by tuning into Cable Network News (CNN) or Headline News (HN). The sitcoms can be replaced by cable's offerings on Home Box Office (HBO) or pay-per-view. ESPN offers sports fare that is never available on the networks (albeit at odd hours). In short, the growth of cable television has given viewers a much greater variety of program choices to suit their tastes.

In health care, a comparable freedom to choose from a wide variety of professionals does not exist. For minor injuries and illnesses, the average American tends to use home remedies first: bandages, ointments, pain relievers, cold medications, cough syrups, etc. However, when faced with illnesses or injuries that are beyond our abilities to treat ourselves, we must go outside the home for our medical care, and this care comes essentially from one source: the doctor.

There are exceptions, which I have already addressed in this book: optometrists, dentists, pharmacists (who can help us with our home medical needs), chiropractors, and in some rural areas that are underserved by physicians, nurse practitioners and physician assistants. Still, the vast majority of our non-home medical treatment is accessed *through* physicians. Please note: I purposely do not say *by* physicians because much of our physician-controlled health care is delivered by nonphysician providers such as nurses, medical technicians, physical therapists, pharmacists, and other allied health practitioners who are following doctors' orders. Little wonder, then, that we automatically think of the doctor when we need health care, just as we used to think of the networks before we got cable.

In America today, the vast majority of our health care is similar to traditional (broadcast) television. There are several network equivalents—the private practice, the hospital emergency room, the free-standing urgent care center (called a "doc in a box" within the trade), the clinic—but they all offer pretty much the same standard service. The professional we see when we tune to any one of these broadcast-channel equivalents is almost always a doctor. We have about as much choice as a television viewer without cable.

As consumers, we should be able to select a health care practitioner based on the provider's *qualified, certified* area of expertise, not just his or her educational degree. A health care professional does not need four years of medical school plus another four years of residency to check a child's ear for infection. Nurse practitioners are an excellent example of alternative health care providers who are capable of treating basic health care needs, and they only require one to two years of specialized training beyond the undergraduate nursing degree.

Health professionals today offer a wide variety of services, and several are capable of expanding their practices to provide greater choices to the public, *if they are so allowed*. In the following pages, I discuss certain allied health professionals who are capable of providing many of the same services as physicians. The remainder of this chapter describes the nursing profession's pursuit of advanced practice skills for independent practice, focusing on two of several paths that nurses have chosen. Chapter 7 presents descriptions of other professionals who have met the standards of independent practice. It also examines ways in which these qualified nonphysician providers can be better utilized in the current health care system and on the barriers that are hindering them from being truly independent. Chapter 8 covers other professions that are still largely dependent on physicians for their orders and discusses new ways in which their skills and knowledge can be used to provide much needed primary care services.

Overall, these three chapters (6, 7, and 8) discuss how each profession meets the basic requirements of independent practice and how each is capable of being the captain of its own ship. Each section presents case scenarios of how these health professionals can be used more effectively to deliver primary care. The scenarios show how health professionals can provide services that were traditionally only handled by physicians. More specifically, the scenarios demonstrate how a medical problem might commonly be treated under the current physician-controlled model and how the treatment might differ if qualified nonphysician providers were allowed to be captains of their own ships. The scenarios are admittedly hypothetical, but they have all been constructed with input from physicians and nonphysicians alike. The fees given in the scenarios are approximations of the charges that my professional sources think would be common under the circumstances. The absolute dollar amounts would be subject to considerable variation, but I have worked to maintain realistic relative relationships between the fees charged under the physician-controlled status quo (the monopoly model) and the competitive possibilities that will hopefully become realities in response to the pressure of consumers who read this book.

The Independent Nurses

For too long, nurses have been considered physicians' handmaidens. Historically, they have been trained to play a supporting role to the doctor in the home, clinic, or hospital. The truth is that the nursing model offers a convincing alternative to the invasive (i.e., surgical) and drug-oriented model of the allopathic physician. Whereas doctors are traditionally trained to "cure," nurses have always been trained to "care." At one time, these functions were not separated; the early physician, lacking the certain ability to cure, had to do both. But as Western medicine gained the power to repair or reverse injury and illness, the curing function was reserved to doctors, and caring was handed over to nurses and other nonphysician providers who followed doctors' orders.

For much of this century, Western medicine has put more emphasis on curing than caring. Yet, by stressing wellness and prevention, caring can minimize the need for cure. Allopathic medicine has made great strides in the twentieth century toward bodily repair, but it has done little (until quite recently, with noteworthy progress in family medicine) in teaching us how to live a healthier life. Nursing, on the other hand, presents a holistic model that looks after the body and mind as a whole, that nurtures health and well-being.

Caring and curing are both integral parts of good health. There is not only room for both, but a *need* for both. This distinction between medicine and nursing (and others like it in the following chapters) is not presented to criticize the medical model, but rather to identify an important difference that ought to be understood by consumers so they can make an intelligent choice of one or the other—or both—depending on their needs and their own concepts of health. Indeed, I am definitely not one of the modern medical reformers who argues that the allopathic model needs to become more holistic. (I do believe the exception to this rule is family practice, a desirable bridge between the two domains that will be explored in more detail in the final chapter.) Specialized allopaths need to spend all their time just keeping up with the curative dimensions of their science. As a medical school professor, I do not see where meaningful instruction on caring could be added to medical specialist's training without taking away from important exposure to the evolving science of curing. As far as I am concerned when I ponder the differences between the various clinical models, *vive la différence!*

Nurse Practitioner

> **Nurse practitioner:** *a nurse who by advanced training and clinical experience in a branch of nursing, as in a master's degree program in nursing, has acquired expert knowledge in a special branch of practice.*[1]

With the medical model justifiably focused on the curing role, the modern nursing model has one more good reason to stand on its own. Nurse practitioners with the right advanced training and experience should be able to practice their special skills without always having to answer to the doctor as "captain of the ship." In states where nurse practitioners have been allowed to practice either independently or under the loose stewardship of a physician, they have demonstrated excellent skills in clinical areas that are ideally suited to the nursing model of caring and wellness. Properly trained nurse practitioners are capable of handling most primary care duties (non-hospital), and even some secondary-care (routine hospital) responsibilities (see sidebar: "Primary, Secondary, and Tertiary Care"). In fact, research shows that many patients prefer nurse practitioners over physicians because nurse practitioners spend more time with the patients, have better listening skills, and educate patients more about their conditions and treatments.[2]

---

1. *Mosby's Medical and Nursing Dictionary*, 2nd edition (St. Louis, C.V. Mosby Company: 1986).
2. Barbara Stilwell, "Different Expectations," *Nursing Times* (June 17, 1987): 59-61.

Primary, Secondary, and Tertiary Care[3]

Primary medical care is the basic level of health services aimed at prevention, early diagnosis, and prompt treatment of disease. It is usually the first point of contact between the patient and the medical care system. Typical primary care services are physical exams; management of common acute illnesses (e.g., pneumonia, sinusitis), management of chronic illness (e.g., high blood pressure), prevention (e.g., pap smears), taking care of minor emergencies (e.g., stitches for simple lacerations), and stabilization of major emergencies (e.g., chest pain). Primary care encompasses approximately 80 percent to 90 percent of all outpatient health care needs.

Secondary care is a more sophisticated, resource-intensive level of health services that requires specialized equipment not commonly found in primary care settings. The patients usually have more severe illnesses (e.g., bacterial meningitis, congestive heart failure, preeclampsia) or injuries (e.g., total hip replacement, compound fracture repair) that require overnight hospitalization, regular testing, and consultations with specialists. Most hospitals today are secondary-care centers.

Tertiary care is the most highly specialized level of medical care. It is offered exclusively in a hospital setting and encompasses the treatment of the most seriously ill or injured patients. Tertiary-care patients typically require longer hospitalizations, extensive testing using the latest technology, and consultations with a wide range of specialists. Patients with rare or complex conditions are typically treated in tertiary-care centers (e.g., pre-term delivery, coronary artery bypass surgery, neurosurgery). Most tertiary-care hospitals are found in urban areas. They require a very large patient base to support and make full use of their high-level skills and technology. Some tertiary-care hospitals attract patients not only from the surrounding areas, but from other states and countries.

---

3. Adopted from *Plugging the Leaks in Health Care: Harnessing Economic Opportunity in Rural America* by Jeffrey C. Bauer, Eileen Weis, and Kimball A. Miller (Denver: Center for the New West, 1992).

Quaternary care is the most advanced form of medical care and is typically reserved for patients who require highly specialized personnel and equipment (e.g., heart-lung and liver transplant surgery, severe burn treatment, reattachment surgery, bone marrow transplants). Quaternary care is conducted in national centers of excellence and usually attracts patients from many states. These centers of excellence typically provide the highest quality of care for certain procedures because of the expertise of their resources and the high volume of patients.

Many people, particularly those who live in states that have not legalized the independent practice of nursing, are unfamiliar with the roles of nurse practitioners. While licensed practical nurses (LPNs) and registered nurses (RNs) are trained to assist in various aspects of giving medical care, nurse practitioners receive extra education and training to be independent providers of medical care. Many hold master's degrees in nursing and specialize in a given clinical area such as family practice, geriatrics, pediatrics, psychiatry, school health, and obstetrics and gynecology. In most states, nurse practitioners are regulated by the state board of nursing, or in a few states, by the state board of nursing and the board of medicine.

Today's nurse practitioners can perform a variety of functions[4]:

1. Obtain medical histories and perform medical examinations.

2. Diagnose and treat common health problems such as infections and minor injuries.

3. Diagnose, treat, and monitor chronic diseases such as diabetes and hypertension.

4. Order and interpret diagnostic tests.

5. Prescribe medicines.

6. Provide prenatal and family planning services.

7. Provide preventive health care through annual physicals, patient education, and counseling.

8. Consult and collaborate with physicians as needed.

4. "The Nurse Practitioner: A Primary Health Care Professional," *American Academy of Nurse Practitioners*, 1994.

In some states, nurse practitioners can already perform as independent contractors, setting up their own practices and using physicians as consultants. Independent nursing practice is a relatively new profession, the result of some of the health care reforms that began in the 1960s in response to the predicted doctor shortage. While programs to educate and train nurse practitioners started with a bang, many of those programs withered away during the later 1970s and throughout the 1980s as a result of funding cuts and physician "disinterest"—another way of saying physicians quite correctly realized that nurse practitioners constituted a competitive threat to their monopoly. The net result is that there are very few nurse practitioners in the United States: 27,226 as of September 1992[5] as compared to approximately 650,000 physicians in 1991.[6]

In spite of the relative scarcity of nurse practitioners, demand for them is increasing, fast. In some areas of the country, in fact, there is an acute shortage. The lack of nurse practitioners has been cited as one of the reasons why rural health clinics, for example, have not achieved their full potential in medically underserved areas.[7] The scenarios interspersed throughout this chapter show why nurse practitioners will likely be in even greater demand as more people recognize the desirable choice that they offer.

Edith

Edith is 70 years old with osteoporosis (brittle bone disease) and chronic hypertension (high blood pressure). Over the past two weeks, she has experienced dizziness on several occasions and mild headaches almost daily. She has put off seeing anyone about it, but she falls during a dizzy spell and decides it's time to get help. She calls her daughter, Diane, who lives 20 miles away, to drive her to the clinic.

5. Walter Morgan, M.D., M.P.H., "Using State Board of Nursing Data to Estimate the Number of Nurse Practitioners in the United States," *Nurse Practitioner* (February 1993): 65-74.
6. U.S. Department of Health and Human Services, January 1992.
7. 1989 Legislative Agenda: A Summary, U.S. House of Representatives, Rural Health Care Collection (March 22, 1989).

Monopoly model: *Diane tells her mother that she can't get off work until after the doctor's office, only open from 9 to 5, will be closed for the day. The visit will have to wait until tomorrow. The next day, Edith is able to get an appointment with a doctor. Diane takes time off from work to drive her mother to the clinic. After waiting 20 minutes, Edith is seen by an internist who determines that Edith's blood pressure is too high and decides to change her medication. At the end of the visit, Edith makes an appointment in the near future to evaluate the effectiveness of the new medication. The total cost of the visit is $40. However, the prescription drug, which is newer than her old medicine and not yet available in generic form, will cost Edith over $50 a month.*

Competitive model: *Diane explains to her mother that she will be over as soon as she gets off work to take her mother to the new clinic, which offers a full range of health care services from both independent nonphysician providers and doctors, and which is open six nights a week. At the clinic, a triage nurse immediately determines that Edith needs to visit with the clinic's geriatric nurse practitioner. Within 10 minutes, the nurse practitioner and Edith are chatting away; they know each other well since Edith has seen the nurse practitioner on other occasions. The nurse practitioner asks Edith about her recent smoking history. Edith confesses that she's still smoking one-half to one pack a day. After measuring Edith's blood pressure and determining it is too high, the nurse practitioner writes a prescription for a new blood pressure medication and discusses with Edith the connection between smoking and hypertension. The NP reminds Edith that her need for medication will be reduced or eliminated if she quits smoking. The NP also strongly encourages Edith to try a smoking cessation class, which Edith then agrees to do. The total cost of the visit is $25, plus $50 a month for the medication.*

Nursing and Independent Practice

Modern nursing in this country began during the Civil War. The battlefield casualties were so great and the bloodshed so horrific that doctors were just too few in number to treat all the wounded. At best, they could treat the acute wounded by digging out bullets or amputating legs, but they hardly had time for ongoing care. Prior to this time, hospitals were generally places where the sick were sent to die, but during the Civil War the Union set up an extensive system of hospitals with the mission of trying to save the wounded. Thanks to the pioneering efforts of a nurse named Florence Nightingale, who demonstrated the life-saving benefits of cleanliness in the hospital setting during the Crimean War, these hospitals for the first time gave the sick or injured a better-than-even chance of coming out alive.

Although nursing made great strides during the latter half of the nineteenth century and the early years of the twentieth, it was left out of the Flexner-era reforms that effectively gave allopathic doctors the monopoly—the power to control patient access to other health professionals. Nursing, of course, was a woman's occupation, and therefore female nurses were subservient to male doctors. But as early as the 1870s, some physicians clearly looked on nurses as possible competitors. As Paul Starr writes:

> Though some doctors approved of the ladies' [New York matron's] desire to establish a nurse's training school, which would attract the wholesome daughters of the middle class, other medical men were opposed. Plainly threatened by the prospect, they objected that educated nurses would not do as they were told—a remarkable comment on the status anxieties of nineteenth century physicians.[8]

The Flexner-era reforms of the early twentieth century only addressed the education of physicians. Nurses were not included. Since the subservient role of nursing was already established by the "captain of the ship" doctrine, medical school reform would presumably trickle down to nursing schools if and when

---

8. Paul Starr, *The Social Transformation of American Medicine*, p. 155.

physicians demanded it. Interestingly enough, medical schools (for men) and nursing schools (for women) bore a greater similarity to each other prior to the changes brought about by Flexner's report than after it; both were vocationally oriented. However, by increasing the length of medical school training and by stressing the general study of science, the Flexner reforms eventually led to the creation of an educated elite and a true profession for the men. Nurses, however, continued to study in vocational schools. This dichotomy between the educated male elite and the vocationally trained female staff further established the doctors' professional dominance over nursing, which was, after all, still only a trade.

This relationship remained essentially unchanged until the 1960s when the convergence of two concepts began to change the role of nurses. The first was the rise of feminism, which empowered nurses to put forward the nursing model as an independent alternative to the allopathic physician model. In short, nurses weren't just the doctors' handmaidens. Empowered by education in women's rights, they began to see nursing as an equally necessary and viable partner in health care. Second, the physician shortage predicted by Rashi Fein gave nursing schools a strong reason to expand their fields of study. They began to move beyond being vocational (trade) schools to becoming true colleges that offered bachelor's, master's, and even doctorate degrees. Many nurses were motivated by a desire to take on more and more of the physicians' functions.

As previously noted, the rapid expansion of these new nursing education programs was relatively short-lived. The perceived "end" of the doctor shortage, coupled with decreased government spending, crippled many advanced nursing programs. Nevertheless, the seed of nursing as a profession was sown, and today many vocationally school-trained nurses go beyond certification to earn college degrees. Indeed, by the end of the 1980s the American Nurses Association had clearly distinguished the professional nurse—one with a four-year college degree in nursing—from the vocational/practical nurses who did not have baccalaureate training.

Julio

Julio, a 38-year old line foreman, is playing basketball at an employee picnic. As he dribbles down court on a fast break, he runs into a defensive player who knocks him hard into the basketball pole. Julio immediately grabs his forearm and sinks to the ground in excruciating pain. The other players run over as he cries, "It feels like it's broken." After about 10 minutes, he allows a few of the men to walk him off the court and into one of their cars so that he can seek medical attention.

Monopoly model: *Julio's buddies immediately take him to a hospital emergency room where he is x-rayed, seen by the emergency room physician, and referred to an orthopedic surgeon. After a physical examination by the orthopedist and an x-ray that identifies a simple fracture, the doctor applies a cast to his arm. His total cost of treatment is $550, which includes the use of the emergency room, x-rays, and consultation by the emergency room physician and orthopedist.*

Competitive model: *Julio's buddies take him to the nurse practitioner clinic three blocks from the ball court. The nurse practitioner examines and x-rays his arm, interprets the x-ray to determine that the fracture is simple, and places a cast on his forearm. The total cost of the visit, $180, includes the examination, x-ray, and cast.*

Despite the professionalization within nursing, it is still perceived by many people to be a dependent rather than an independent health profession. After all, ships need crews, and nursing has more than proven itself to be an able supplier of high-quality assistance for physicians. Licensed practical nurses (LPNs) with one to two years of technical training and diploma registered nurses (RNs) with two to three years of apprenticeship still comprise the majority of all nurses. Now, however, LPNs and RNs have the option to continue their education to earn a Bachelor of Science degree in Nursing (BSN), a Master of Science degree in Nursing (MSN), or a Ph.D.

The primary focus of nursing education at all levels, unlike medical school education, continues to be patient care rather than diagnosis and treatment of specific conditions. Particularly at the masters and doctoral levels, nurses are generally expected to conduct research that applies to the advancement of the nursing profession, not medical science *per se*. Some nurses continue to pursue advanced clinical work; many within this group become nurse practitioners. Others choose to concentrate on administrative or educational functions, which will qualify them to run clinics and hospitals or to teach future nurses.

Clearly, nurses who choose to continue their education and training toward advanced degrees and certification can also meet the other six foundations of professional autonomy. Like doctors, nurses subscribe to the scientific base on which Western medicine is built. Similarly, nurses follow a coherent clinical model, adhere to a strong professional ethic, are willing and able to accept professional liability, and are subject to standards of quality control equal to physicians. They qualify to be captains of their own ships, to provide an alternative to the good—but different—ship, "U.S.S. Allopathic Medicine."

Properly trained and certified nurse practitioners have ample training to manage their own primary care practices. They are probably the most cost-effective resource for meeting our nation's shortage of primary care providers. I do not argue that nurses should replace primary care physicians, merely that they provide a competitive alternative and a different approach to basic health care. (A funny thing happened on the way to solving the doctor shortage; the vast majority of the new doctors went into specialties. Now, everyone agrees we have a serious primary care shortage, which I will address in my concluding chapter.)[9]

---

9. Indeed, in one of my last acts as chief planning officer at the University of Colorado Health Sciences Center, I argued in 1984 that our medical school should be converted totally to the education of primary-care doctors. This proposal enraged some of my medical school colleagues and accelerated my decision to become a self-employed medical economist and health futurist.

Susan

Susan's three-year-old daughter, Amy, has had a recurring history of earaches and ear infections. To confuse the matter, Amy's frequent complaint, "My ear hurts, Mommy," is sometimes a false alarm. To Susan, hauling Amy to the doctor is a hit-or-miss proposition. Sometimes there appears to be a clinical cause for the problem, sometimes not. While Susan's employer supplies major medical insurance, the family must still pay the first $1,000 worth of care. Amy wakes up one Saturday morning after a fitful night, complaining that her ear aches. Since Amy appeared to be coming down with a cold on Friday, Susan suspects a true ear infection.

Monopoly model: Susan calls her family doctor's office and is referred by the telephone answering service to a large local medical clinic for an "emergency appointment." She phones the clinic, and a nurse tells her to come in before noon when the clinic closes. Susan takes Amy to the clinic, where Susan fills out the appropriate forms covering Amy's medical history. After waiting 45 minutes, mother and daughter are ushered into an examination room where a nurse takes Amy's temperature and asks how she feels. They wait 10 minutes longer until the doctor arrives. He quickly examines Amy's throat, ears, and nostrils and feels under her jaw for any swelling of the lymph glands. "Yes, there is a bit of an infection just beginning here," he pronounces. Before going on to his next patient, he quickly writes a prescription and hands it to Susan, telling her to check back with her family physician in 10 days. The length of his entire visit is about five minutes. The charge for the examination is $50, plus a $35 "emergency care" charge for a Saturday appointment; the total is $85.

Competitive model: Susan takes Amy to a local shopping center with a variety of stores, including a grocery, pharmacy, dry cleaner, restaurant, some specialty shops, and a neighborhood *clinic. Like the grocery store next door, the clinic is open 24 hours a day, seven days a week. When Susan and Amy walk in, they are immediately recognized by the triage nurse, who has a daughter who goes to Amy's school. "Hello, Amy. Do you have another earache?" she asks. Amy nods. Susan and Amy take a seat in the reception area. Within five minutes they are ushered into an examination room. A nurse practitioner arrives shortly with a computerized printout of Amy's medical history. She introduces herself, saying, "You usually see Mr. Ryan, I see." She further explains that she is new to the clinic, but she has had a chance to get to know Mr. Ryan, another nurse practitioner on the staff. She examines Amy's throat, ears, and nostrils, and checks the lymph glands under Amy's jaw. "Looks like you have the beginnings of an ear infection," she says, and writes a prescription. Then she turns to Susan. "I see from Amy's chart that she has had a lot of ear infections. Mr. Ryan has noted that various causes ought to be explored. I would suggest you call him on Monday to talk about having Amy tested for certain allergies." Susan says she will, and thanks the nurse practitioner. Susan and Amy are in and out of the neighborhood clinic within half an hour. The total cost of the visit is $25.*

I believe that converting several existing medical schools to centers of excellence in training only primary care physicians—including the retraining of oversupplied specialists who are already in practice—would be a very good idea. Creating several Schools of Primary care Medicine would be the most cost-effective response to our nation's unmet needs for primary care doctors because it would capture economies of scale in medical education, and it would eliminate the loss of primary care doctors to medical specialties because specialty training would not be available to students in these schools. A substantial reward should be made available for the first medical school that voluntarily redirects all its resources to training only primary care doctors.

However, reorienting medical education will not meet all our needs or give us all the choices we deserve. Nursing schools are much less expensive than medical schools, and nurses require fewer years of education to become competent in basic primary care. Therefore, training more nurse practitioners will give us an even greater and faster return on future investments in primary care education. The lower cost of nurse practitioner education has another significant advantage: nurse practitioners enter practice with much less educational debt than doctors. They do not need to charge high fees to recoup high educational costs by earning high incomes; they can afford to be a cost-effective competitor.

Furthermore, nursing education emphasizes caring for the whole person, not repairing body parts. The net result of opening the health care system to independent nurse practitioners will be lower primary care costs and a greater emphasis on wellness and prevention. In the long run, a less-expensive primary care system emphasizing wellness and prevention will also mean lower secondary and tertiary medical costs because more conditions will be "nipped in the bud" or prevented altogether. Lower, more competitive primary care costs will also make health services accessible to more people who might otherwise wait to seek medical care until an illness or injury becomes serious—and thus more expensive in both monetary and human terms. The added competition will not force doctors to reduce the quality of their service, but it will put some price pressure on doctors' charges. Lowering the costs of health care is a primary objective of health care reform, but accomplishing the goal through competition is a whole lot more promising than doing it through the untried and complex schemes currently being discussed in Washington.

If nurse practitioners were used to their full potential in the United States, the annual cost savings to the health care system has been estimated to be somewhere between $6.4 billion and $8.75 billion.[10] But nurse practitioners and their other advanced-practice colleagues—nurse midwives and nurse anesthetists—are not always "utilized adequately because of significant barriers to their practice in the areas of legal scope of practice, reimbursement, and prescriptive authority. These barriers of practice vary in severity from state to

---

10. The information in this paragraph is from Linda J. Pearson, "1992-1993 Update: How Each State Stands on Legislative Issues Affecting Advanced Nursing Practice," *Nurse Practitioner* (January 1993): 23-27.

state." For example, even though NPs can prescribe medicines in 45 states (including the District of Columbia), the extent of their prescriptive authority varies. Some advanced-practice nurses must have a physician's signature on prescriptions, while NPs in other states do not. Approximately 40 states allow for independent prescriptive authority, in which physician signatures on prescription pads are not necessary. In this arrangement, NPs have greater freedom to practice in a style that is safer and more convenient to themselves and to their patients. Regarding the important issue of reimbursement, health insurance companies are required to pay for nurse practitioners' services in several states, but many states do not require direct payment to the NP. Thirty-eight states reported that advanced-practice nurses receive some form of private third-party reimbursement. However, only 24 states have legislatively mandated private third-party reimbursement to NPs.

Under government-financed health insurance programs, 42 states permit Medicaid reimbursement for NPs at rates ranging from 85 percent to 100 percent of a physician's Medicaid payment for the same service. "Medicare covers the services of NPs in nursing homes, rural areas, rural health clinics, health maintenance organizations, federally qualified health centers (FQHCs) and ambulatory care settings when the service is 'incident to' a physician's service."[11] The rural-area provisions are the only direct-reimbursement provisions under Medicare.

Comparison of Mean Annual Incomes	
Family Physician, 1991	$101,160[12]
Nurse Practitioner, 1993	$50,000[13]
Source: American Academy of Nurse Practitioners,[12] Medical Economics[13]	

11. Pamela C. Mittelstadt, "Federal Reimbursement of Advanced Practice Nurses' Services Empowers the Profession," *Nurse Practitioner,* (January 1993): 43-49.
12. Linda Walsh and Jeanne DeJoseph, "Findings of the 1991 Annual American College of Nurse-Midwives Membership Survey," *Journal of Nurse-Midwifery,* vol. 38, no. 1, (January/February 1993): 38.
13. Arthur Owens, "What's the Recession Done to Your Buying Power?" *Medical Economics,* (September 7, 1992): 197.

Educating the Public

At my local health facility, East Morgan County Hospital in Brush, Colorado, the first nurse practitioner (NP) was hired in 1993 to work in the hospital's primary care clinic. While the hospital administration knew that the new nurse practitioner would deliver safe and appropriate care, the community had absolutely no prior experience with an NP and did not know what to expect. Therefore, the administration was not certain that the community would use the NP enough to justify her salary.

With this concern in mind, the hospital embarked on an ambitious promotional campaign. It placed display advertisements in the local newspaper to describe nurse practitioners in general and the new NP in particular. Each patient who had an appointment to see the NP was given a detailed descriptive brochure upon arrival at the clinic. By the time the NP came into the exam room, each patient already knew something about NPs and how they are different from doctors.

The brochures, newspaper advertisements, and word-of-mouth advertising were so effective that the new nurse practitioner was fully booked within two months. Many patients were asking to see her directly, not one of the physicians. The promotional campaign, intended to last at least six months, was terminated and plans were immediately made to hire another NP. Thanks to a successful promotional campaign and very positive initial experiences with the NP, the town went from knowing nothing about nurse practitioners to wanting another one in just two months.

Mandated direct reimbursement is necessary for NPs to have a financially viable practice, and it also makes them more attractive to patients who prefer to have their insurance—not themselves—pay for their care. Fighting against direct reimbursement is an effective way that doctors can hinder the competition, even after state laws have granted the right of independent practice to nonphysician providers. Consequently, specific provisions for direct reimbursement need to be included in plans to bring much-needed competition to the medical care delivery system.

Insurance companies ought to be strongly supportive of mandated reimbursement for nurse practitioners, so any resistance to the principle is a potential sign of influence from a monopoly that is trying to protect its market power. Because nurse practitioners cost less overall—as shown by the income differential in the sidebar above and the actual fee differences in the scenarios— third-parties can save money when they pay an NP rather than an MD for a comparable primary care service. (Indeed, this principle is the foundation of one of the four steps of the action plan in the last chapter.) When operating independently, nurse practitioners are currently able to offer standard primary care services for lower fees than physicians. *No wonder, then, that price-sensitive payers, including patients who pay out-of-pocket for such services, are interested in being able to purchase routine care directly from a nurse practitioner.* If physicians are threatened by the competition, maybe they will lower their fees.

Certified Nurse Midwife

> **Certified Nurse Midwife:** *registered nurse qualified by advanced training in obstetric and neonatal care and certified by the American College of Nurse Midwives. The nurse midwife manages the perinatal care of women having a normal pregnancy, labor, and childbirth.*[14]

Like nurse practitioners, certified nurse midwives provide an attractive alternative to the traditional obstetrics and gynecology model of allopathic medicine. Many women prefer a certified nurse midwife (CNM) to a traditional obstetrician because they feel that the CNM is more sensitive to their needs and will work harder to ensure that prenatal care and childbirth are as natural as possible.

---

14. *Mosby's Medical and Nursing Dictionary*, 2nd edition (St. Louis: C.V. Mosby Company, 1986).

Many people don't realize that midwives predate physicians by many millennia as the primary caregivers for women and birthing. In fact, in the western world midwives provided care for most female needs (including childbirth) until the mid- or late-nineteenth century, and they are still responsible for childbirth in most of the rest of the world. The shift of responsibility from lay midwives to physicians began in Europe about 450 years ago, but it was only "completed" in this country within the past half-century. Many reasons have been given to explain this shift. Midwives' early competitors were the barber-surgeons, who at the time were separate from physicians. The barber-surgeons were closer to the lowly midwives on the social scale, and both were substantially beneath the university-trained physicians. The barber-surgeons actually did provide a function different from midwives; in complicated births barber-surgeons, who were not afraid to use a scalpel, offered another method of saving mother or child, or even both. Gradually, barber-surgeons began taking over a greater number of midwife functions.

By the middle of the nineteenth century, surgery had been embraced by physicians as an acceptable medical practice. With that acceptance, the two once separate disciplines—medicine and surgery—began to merge into a single profession. Physicians had already established themselves in obstetrics, and in fact were attracting more and more middle-class and upper-class patients by virtue of their advanced education. This trend continued in the United States so that:

> by the twentieth century, male physicians had become the "authorities" on health. They had led a successful campaign during the late nineteenth and early twentieth centuries to eliminate midwives and sharply reduce the number of female physicians. For the first time in the history of the world, women were forbidden by law to be responsible for other women's childbirths, and were replaced almost exclusively by male physicians.[15]

Nevertheless, midwives still had a role in catering to the poor and women living outside more heavily populated areas. In fact, a program to certify nurse midwives began in the 1920s for women practicing in the Frontier Nursing

15. From "The Politics of Women and Medical Care" by Hilary Salk, Wendy Sanford, Norman Swenson, and Judith Dickson Luce, published in The Boston Women's Health Book Collective, *The New Our Bodies, Ourselves* (New York: Touchstone, 1992) p. 657. This source provides an excellent discussion on the history of women and the medical profession.

Service and Maternity Care Association,[16] and as many as 40,000 to 50,000 midwives still practiced in the United States as late as 1930.[17] While lay midwives all but disappeared by the mid-1960s, the profession of *certified nurse midwife* (CNM), professionally trained and educated in the latest obstetric practices, began to attract more and more women in the nursing field for reasons I have already mentioned: 1) the nonphysician health care field was growing at this time; 2) Medicare and Medicaid created a sudden demand for more health care providers because of the predicted doctor shortage; and 3) women were developing a strong awareness of women's issues.

Like other nonphysician providers seeking autonomy, certified nurse midwives have been greeted with ambivalence by doctors. On the one hand, the CNMs have been encouraged to practice in "underserved" areas (that is, areas where physicians do not wish to go) such as inner cities and rural counties. On the other hand, CNMs are frequently denied the privileges to work in many urban hospitals. In most states, certified nurse midwives are allowed to practice independently as long as they can find a physician for back-up. But in some states, such as Colorado, very few certified nurse midwives have practiced in the past because doctors are unwilling to work with them (another subtle monopoly ploy—legalize the competition as long as it works with you, then refuse to provide the necessary support).

In those areas where the services of a certified nurse midwife are available, many women either are unaware that this option exists or believe that no nonphysician provider could possibly be as competent as a physician. While we can be pleased that more and more women are becoming doctors and that a relatively large percentage of them are specializing in obstetrics and family practice, they are still being educated in the traditional allopathic world of the medical schools. Unlike the obstetrician/gynecologists and family-practice physicians who deliver babies, certified nurse midwives are trained in the complementary disciplines of nursing and midwifery (that is, care of the pregnant woman and childbirth) and thus offer the expectant mother a more supportive and holistic alternative—one with minimal reliance on drugs and surgical intervention.

---

16. Jane Pincus, "Pregnancy" in The Boston Women's Health Book Collective *The New Our Bodies, Ourselves*, p. 410.
17. Rosemary Stevens, *American Medicine and the Public Interest*, p. 180.

Joan

Shortly after her 28th birthday, Joan discovers she is pregnant for the first time. Because she and her husband Mike have just recently moved to a new city, she does not currently have a health care practitioner for normal gynecological care. She realizes that she must seek professional assistance for her pregnancy.

Monopoly model: Joan asks several friends and co-workers to recommend a good obstetrician. After interviewing two physicians, she chooses one to handle the pregnancy. Her pregnancy progresses normally, and Joan and her husband attend the traditional birthing classes. But the baby is late and Joan becomes nervous. One week after the expected delivery date, labor finally begins. After eleven hours in a hospital birthing room and with Joan's consent, the obstetrician performs a cesarean section, delivering a healthy boy. The total cost of the delivery, including a five-day stay in the hospital and physician fees, is $8,000.

Competitive model: Joan interviews several obstetricians and nurse midwives, ultimately selecting a certified nurse midwife for prenatal care and delivery. During the pregnancy, Joan and her husband attend the traditional birthing classes. In addition, the nurse midwife, who has had two children of her own, recommends that Joan take some special childbirth preparation classes that incorporate methods of relaxation and breathing. Rather than having her baby in a hospital, Joan chooses to deliver in a birthing clinic nearby. While the clinic is staffed by nurse practitioners, there is an obstetrician on-premise eight hours a day, and on-call 24 hours a day. One week after Joan's expected due date, labor begins. The labor lasts longer than expected—a full eleven hours—but due to her extensive training in natural childbirth, Joan is finally able to vaginally deliver a healthy baby boy. The total cost of delivery and a 23-hour stay in the birthing clinic is $2,300, which includes the nurse midwife's charges.

I have heard some proponents of midwifery advance the argument that nurse midwives approach birth as a celebration, whereas physicians approach it as a disease. While I think this position is unfair to many doctors who deliver babies, I do note with some sadness that this fundamentally natural part of life has moved out of the everyday setting of wellness—the home—into the one place in America reserved for sick people—the hospital—since physicians took control over birthing. Less than a century ago, only one in every 20 babies was born in a hospital; today only one in every 20 is not.[18]

Foreigners have great difficulty believing that almost all American babies are delivered by doctors in hospitals. In most other developed countries, babies are commonly delivered by midwives in maternal clinics or in the home. Other countries also have fewer cesarean sections and episiotomies and impressively lower infant mortality rates.

The philosophical difference between nurse midwives and doctors might be appropriately summarized by contrasting questions that reflect the clinical paradigm of each. Physicians ask, "How can I (the doctor) prevent anything from going *wrong* with the pregnancy and birth?" Nurse midwives ask, "How can we (the expectant mother, her family, and the practitioner) make everything go *right*?"

Comparison of Mean Annual Incomes, 1991	
Obstetrician	$198,380[19]
Certified Nurse Midwife	$50,446[20]
Source: Journal of Nurse-Midwifery,[19] *Medical Economics*[20]	

---

18. From "Childbirth." by Jane Pincus and Norma Swenson. In *The New Our Bodies, Ourselves,* p. 438.
19. Linda Walsh and Jeanne DeJoseph, "Findings of the 1991 Annual American College of Nurse-Midwives Membership Survey," *Journal of Nurse-Midwifery,* vol. 38, no. 1, (January/February 1993): 38.
20. Arthur Owens, "What's the Recession Done to Your Buying Power?" *Medical Economics,* (September 7, 1992): 197.

Tamara

Tamara is 16, the oldest of four children, and a good student at her inner-city high school. Unfortunately, she discovers she's pregnant. She's afraid to tell her mom, Rita, who works hard as a grocery clerk in order to support the family. (Tamara's dad has long since disappeared.) After much thought, she decides that she wants to keep the baby. She finally breaks the news to her mom, who is initially dismayed but eventually supports her daughter's decision.

Monopoly model: Unfortunately, Rita does not have health insurance to cover Tamara's pregnancy. Nevertheless, she takes her daughter to the doctor, who confirms the pregnancy and tells Tamara to come back once a month for prenatal checkups. Rita pays the $60 bill for the checkup and the test. Rita and Tamara skip the first two checkups because of the cost. In the fifth month of pregnancy, Tamara goes into premature labor. Rita takes her daughter to the hospital. By the time Tamara is able to see a doctor, it is too late to stop the labor, and Tamara gives birth to a three-pound, eight-ounce baby girl. The baby is immediately rushed to the hospital's premature infant unit, where doctors and nurses struggle to keep it alive. Tamara suffers some minor complications with the delivery but recovers within a few days. The baby is kept in the hospital for several weeks. The total cost of the labor, delivery, hospital care for mother, and intensive care for the baby is $30,000. Rita is only able to pay about one-third of the cost over a period of five years.

Competitive model: Rita has been taking her family to a local clinic staffed by nonphysician providers for several years now. One of the optional benefits she receives from her employment is a "wellness" membership in the clinic. For a fixed annual cost, deducted each week from her paycheck, she and her family receive all their outpatient medical services from the clinic, subject to a $10 co-pay per visit. The clinic offers free classes on self-care, *and even has a small gym and exercise room where members can work out. Rita and Tamara visit the nurse midwife at the clinic, who confirms the pregnancy. The nurse practitioner enrolls Tamara in a "teen mom" class where Tamara learns about proper care for herself and her future baby. On Tamara's third visit to the nurse midwife, about four months into the pregnancy, a problem is discovered through an ultrasound examination. The nurse midwife immediately consults with an obstetrician/gynecologist associated with the clinic. They agree to put Tamara on a medication to lower the possibility of premature labor. The nurse midwife prescribes the medication for Tamara, tells her to slow down on her activities, and counsels her on what to do if she does go into labor early. Four months later, Tamara is feeling tired and run down. She wakes up one morning to discover she's been bleeding vaginally. She calls up her nurse midwife and describes her symptoms. The nurse midwife tells her to get to the hospital immediately. Tamara takes a cab, and the nurse midwife meets her in the emergency room. After a thorough examination, including a number of tests, the nurse midwife decides that both Tamara and the fetus are in danger. She recommends surgical intervention. An hour later, the clinic's consulting obstetrician/gynecologist delivers Tamara's healthy baby girl via cesarean section. Rita's insurance through her employer covers all but $1,000 of Tamara's doctor and hospital bill. Since Tamara gave birth to a healthy baby, there are no additional charges for the child.*

I do not argue that certified nurse midwives should replace obstetricians. They are both competent professionals in their own right, and each makes a distinctly valuable contribution to medical care. CNMs are trained for low-risk birthing situations, which constitute a substantial portion of all births in the United States. Obstetricians, with their advanced training in the potential complications of the birthing process, can and should deal with "problem" pregnancies and other high-risk births. I believe the argument is strong, however, that in low-risk cases CNMs could be better prepared than the typical family doctor to care for the expectant mother and the childbirth process because childbirth is all midwives do. A growing body of published reports suggests convincingly that the quality of a provider's care is directly proportional to the frequency with which the care is provided. For example, heart surgeons who perform a given procedure hundreds of times a year achieve much better patient outcomes than heart surgeons who perform the procedure only a few dozen times. The same relationship is likely to hold in the case of performing low-risk births, lending strong support for policies to promote the CNM as a competitive alternative to the family doctor for low-risk pregnancies.

Specialization has arisen within the allopathic medical model for good reason. Medical science has expanded our knowledge of ever more minute aspects of human health, correspondingly requiring doctors to become more specialized because they, like the rest of us, have a limited number of hours in a day to keep up with their clinical areas. (I am reminded of the old aphorism about narrowly focused academicians who are said to keep learning more and more about less and less until they know everything about nothing.) Marcus Welby no longer exists because no doctor today can possibly know everything there is to know about all of medicine. In this regard, a certified nurse midwife and an obstetrician/gynecologist have more in common than an obstetrician/gynecologist and a family practitioner: The CNM and the "ob/gyn" are both *specialists* in women's care and childbirth, whereas most general or family practitioners by definition are not.

Certified nurse midwifes are registered nurses who have advanced training in obstetrics and gynecology (frequently at the master's level) and become nationally certified through the American College of Nurse-Midwives (ACNM). In addition, they must meet specific state requirements such as licensure to practice midwifery. Whether operating under the "umbrella" of a physician or as independent practitioners, CNMs can provide prenatal care, labor and delivery management, postpartum care, well-woman gynecology, and normal newborn care. CNMs are also authorized to prescribe specific drugs and treatments to patients in at least 36 states, as of 1991.[21]

---

21. "Report on Nurse-Midwifery Legislation," *Journal of Nurse-Midwifery*, vol. 37, no. 3, (May/June 1992): 206-209.

But remember not to be fooled by impressive statistics that might seem to suggest CNMs are available in most states; they are hardly available at all in some states where they are perfectly legal because doctors are subtly able to suppress the competition. Despite midwifery's long history of caring for women and newborns, only about 4,000 certified midwives are practicing in this country today. A large number of positions in both urban and rural areas are left vacant because there are simply not enough nurse midwives to fill them even if physicians were not an impediment. Part of the shortage is due to the overall decline in enrollment in nursing programs, which feed the nurse midwifery programs.[22] Another reason is the high cost of malpractice insurance, which can sometimes be one-third of the typical CNM salary. The insurance crisis indirectly encourages CNMs to spurn independent practice in favor of working directly for hospitals or physicians because larger organizations will frequently pay their malpractice insurance.

CNMs also have an incentive to work for physicians in states with requirements that CNMs must have a supervising physician. Some states interpret that to be a physician "on site," which is often impractical in many situations (e.g., remote rural areas, areas with physician shortages) because physicians may not be available. The standard regulations typically call for physicians to be available for consultation and referral, which means they can be located in another town.

Limited access to hospital privileges is a continuing problem for CNMs. Many hospital boards prohibit CNMs from using their birthing rooms or labor and delivery rooms unless they are directly employed by a physician or the hospital. In other words, hospital policies—not state laws—can limit CNMs' ability to manage labor and births as independent practitioners. Most hospital boards will take a stand against giving hospital privileges to independent nurse midwives after consulting with their medical staffs because doctors do not want competition. Opposition, of course, comes in the form of physicians raising subtle questions about the ability of CNMs to handle emergency situations or birth complications beyond their training. "Why not have an ob/gyn handle the birth in the first place," the doctors argue, "just in case something should

---

22. R. Lichtman, "More Voices for Educational Innovation," *Journal of Nurse-Midwifery*, (January/February 1990): 1-2.

go wrong?" The hospital boards would get very different advice if they were to talk instead to women who were informed of the alternatives.

Just like many other allied health professionals, CNMs must fight in their state legislatures to establish or preserve mandated insurance reimbursement. There is no question that the ability of CNMs to practice independently is enhanced once direct reimbursement is mandated, so states can foster the development of independent CNM practices by ensuring direct and mandatory reimbursement. At least 26 states mandated private insurance reimbursement of CNMs as of 1992.[23]

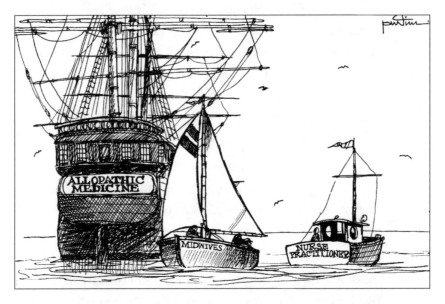

Insurance companies are also known to fight against mandated reimbursement of CNMs so that they will not have to incur the costs of administering benefits for yet another group of professionals. While these arguments carry weight in predominantly male and politically conservative state legislatures, strong evidence suggests that women with a healthy pregnancy, labor, and delivery are just as safe with a certified nurse midwife as with a physician. The quality of care provided by certified nurse midwives is equivalent to that provided by physicians for low-risk pregnancies.[24]

---

23. "Report on Nurse-Midwifery Legislation," *Journal of Nurse-Midwifery*, vol. 37, no. 3, (May/June 1992): 206-209.
24. United State Congress, Office of Technology Assessment, "Nurse Practitioners, Physicians Assistants, and Certified Nurse-Midwives: A Policy Analysis" (Washington, DC: U.S. Government Printing Office, 1986): 5-6.

Juanita

Juanita, her husband Roberto, and their two children live in a small coastal community that has a failing hospital and a doctor shortage. Roberto has worked at a steady job in landscaping, but he earns only slightly more than minimum wage and receives no insurance benefits. Despite efforts to avoid having more children, Juanita discovers she is pregnant again. She is able to receive prenatal care through a local public clinic but is told that she must have the baby delivered at a county hospital in a large city 50 miles away. There used to be two obstetricians in the town where Juanita and her family live, but they moved to larger cities five years ago. And the town's family practice physicians (one of whom delivered her first two children) have stopped delivering babies due to the added cost of malpractice insurance for obstetric care.

Monopoly model: When Juanita feels the onset of labor, she calls her husband, who leaves work to drive her the 50 miles to the county hospital. Fortunately, all goes smoothly, and Juanita delivers a healthy baby girl. The cost for the delivery and one-night stay in the hospital is $2,000 and the physician fee is $1,300, for a total of $3,300. Juanita and her husband eventually pay the hospital bill over a period of five years.

Competitive model: Juanita decides to use a certified nurse midwife located in her home town for the management of her pregnancy and delivery. Roberto and Juanita attend birthing classes, the pregnancy proceeds normally, and Juanita delivers a baby girl at a birthing clinic attached to a nurse practitioner's office. Fortunately, the total for all services is less than $1,400. Roberto and Juanita are able to pay off the entire bill before their new daughter turns two.

Further, "certified nurse midwives are more adept than physicians at providing services that depend on communication with patients and preventive actions . . . Patients are generally satisfied with the quality of care provided by . . . CNMs, particularly with the interpersonal aspects of care."[25] Cost effectiveness studies indicate that the average hospital bill for patients who used certified nurse midwives was $114 less than the average bill for patients who used physicians.[26] Another study demonstrated a significantly lower rate of cesarean births at a maternity center staffed with certified nurse midwives than at a university hospital staffed with physicians and residents. In other words, research has demonstrated that CNMs are less likely than physicians to have babies delivered via cesarean section.[27]

The Institute of Medicine is a significant medical organization that recommends greater use of CNMs. In a paper on preventing low birth weight, the Institute proposes that "more reliance be placed on nurse-midwives . . . to increase access to prenatal care for hard-to-reach, often high-risk groups." The paper adds that "certified nurse-midwives . . . have been shown to be particularly effective in managing the care of pregnant women who are at high risk of low birth weight because of social and economic factors." The Institute also supports the use of nurse midwives because of the "difficulty in some communities of finding physicians willing to work in public clinics or with low-income women."[28]

While this endorsement of certified nurse midwives is welcomed, I wonder if it would be as strong—or if it would even exist—if CNMs were competing directly with physicians in more affluent areas where third-party resources pay for most patient care. To me, the bottom line is this: if nurse midwives are acknowledged to be fully competent within their defined scope of practice—a scope of practice that covers the majority of births in this country—then they should be allowed to practice in all markets, not just areas where physicians

---

25. The American College of Nurse-Midwives Fact Sheet.
26. Donna Diers and Helen Varney Burst, "Effectiveness of Policy Related Research: Nurse-Midwifery as Case Study," Nurse-Midwifery (Summer 1983): 68 supra.
27. Gigliola Baruffi, Donna Strobino, and Lisa Payne, "Investigation of Institutional Differences in Primary Cesarean Birth Rates, Journal of Nurse-Midwifery, vol., 35, no. 5 (September/October 1990): 274-281.
28. "Preventing Low Birthweight: Summary," Institute of Medicine, (Washington, D.C., National Academy Press 1985): 25.

are in short supply. Indeed, as a real rural resident (try finding Hillrose, Colorado, on a map!), I resent patronizing health policies based on the implicit belief that "second-best" solutions are acceptable in areas that do not have enough doctors. If some professional is not good enough for the city, we rural folk don't want him or her our here, either. In other words, I do not see any special rural or city-center dimension to the arguments in favor of allowing independent practice to qualified nonphysicians. The medical monopoly is a problem for our entire country, not just for medically underserved areas.

Women and their families need a high-quality, cost-competitive alternative to the traditional allopathic (and usually male) doctor who provides gynecological and obstetrical services. Like many other allied health practitioners capable of independent practice, certified nurse midwives are a profession ready to fill that need. We need to remove the anticompetitive barriers that keep them out of the market.

Chapter Seven

Other Independent Providers

The fact that some clinical specialties broke away from allopathic medicine and others did not is more a function of historical accident than of any logical plan. For example, why are dentists educated in dental schools and awarded DMD or DDS degrees? Why don't they go to medical school instead and get the MD degree, followed by a residency in medicine of the mouth? Why do podiatrists have their own medical colleges and their own degree, the DPM, even though orthopedic surgeons provide virtually all the same services? And why did optometrists—trained in schools of optometry—evolve as a competitive alternative to ophthalmologists who are trained in medical schools?

The answers to these questions seem to be a function of at least two variables: 1) when the evolution of the disciplines occurred; and 2) whether the members of the nonphysician group were able to stand up to (and exist separately from) the allopathic physician monopoly as it became established during the early part of this century. The largely independent existence of these similar professions also disproves any allopathic claims that the quality of patient care is diminished when qualified nonphysicians gain their independence from mainstream medicine.

As I have noted throughout this book, many competitive alternatives to physicians did not survive at all outside the allopathic sphere. Others managed to maintain at least some degree of independence—but not always total autonomy because physicians still maintained control over important parts of the discipline. This chapter examines health professions that have established some autonomy, showing both the creation of successful competition and work yet to be done.

Optometrist

> **Optometrist:** *person trained in testing the eyes for visual acuity, prescribing corrective lenses, and recommending eye exercises.*[1]

Ophthalmology has been a subspecialty of medicine since the eighteenth century, perhaps even before. Specialized eye clinics began in the nineteenth century, and many advancements in eye care were made in that 100-year span. It is generally believed that legitimate ophthalmologists had to compete with a broad range of quacks during this era. At the same time, opticians were dispensing glasses to those who needed them, often apart from medical doctors who were more interested in diseases of the eye than in optical correction. This led to an inevitable "turf battle" as doctors began to claim that eye examinations and prescriptions should be left to them rather than to the lowly and often ill-trained optician.[2] After failure of an attempt to set the same standards for both ophthalmologists and opticians, optometry evolved as a profession different from either.[3] Physicians laid claim to ophthalmology—and therefore the ability to perform surgery and prescribe medicine. Optometrists secured the right to administer eye exams and write corrective lens prescriptions. The opticians were left to grind the lenses and fit the corrective eye wear.

---

1. *Mosby's Medical and Nursing Dictionary*, 2nd edition, (St. Louis: C.V. Mosby Company 1986).
2. Stevens, *American Medicine and the Public Interest*, p. 103.
3. Stevens, *American Medicine and the Public Interest*, pp. 106-107.

Abe

At 71, Abe is in pretty good health. He is fit, not overweight, and never needed to wear glasses. But for the past several years, he's had trouble seeing things that are not directly in front of him. Though his family has suspected the problem, it's never really been discussed. One afternoon, while driving his daughter and two grandchildren to a shopping mall, he runs into another car which, he says, he "just didn't see." His daughter decides it's time he had his vision checked.

Monopoly model: Abe makes an appointment with an M.D. ophthalmologist who diagnoses his narrowing of peripheral vision as glaucoma and prescribes special eye drops. The cost of the physician visit, including a complete eye exam, is $61, and the medication is $25.

Competitive model: Abe visits an optometrist who has been certified to diagnose and treat specific types of eye disease that do not require surgical intervention. The optometrist recognizes Abe's narrowing of peripheral vision as glaucoma and prescribes the necessary eye drops. The total cost of the visit is $41, and the eye drops are $25.

Since then, optometry has made significant gains and has largely established itself as a good example of the model I am proposing for all professions that meet the foundations of independent clinical practice. Optometrists practice independently—that is, they can see patients directly without those patients having to visit a physician first—and they are reimbursed for their services by both patients and third-party payers. Consequently, new optometry graduates are being prepared to practice in this more permissive environment by studying pharmacology and disease management in school. As a result, optometrists can now treat about 90 percent of all eye problems, proving to be able practitioners of primary care.[4] However, they still do not have the authority to perform surgery on the eye and are denied prescriptive privileges in many states.

4. Dr. James Leadingham, president of the American Optometric Association and faculty member at the Southern College of Optometry. Personal interview (March 3, 1993).

A growing number of states now allow optometrists to use and prescribe both diagnostic and therapeutic pharmaceuticals. Thus, many optometrists can now administer certain antibiotics and antivirals for specific eye disorders. But their ability to freely use medication is still subject to state laws, which tend to vary in their restrictiveness. For example, in California, optometrists are allowed to use drugs to diagnose but not to treat—even though diagnostic drugs are perceived to be more dangerous than those used in treatment.

Despite these advances, recently trained optometrists and those with specific continuing education believe they can go further, even toward treating certain diseases of the eye like glaucoma (an eye disease that results in blindness) and iritis (inflamed part of the eye). Other optometrists are interested in acquiring the skills to use laser therapy. With special light lasers, they can remove certain types of eye scars and treat eye disorders resulting from diabetes, perform corneal sculpting to eliminate the need for glasses (different from radial keratotomy, a more invasive procedure), and perform treatments after cataract surgery. However, optometrists will have to fight on a legislative level, as they have successfully done before, to legally acquire the rights to perform these practices.

Ophthalmologists are still generally inclined to protect their turf by opposing optometrists' efforts to gain authority to provide skills that have been solely in the domain of medical doctors. As optometry expands its capabilities in the noninvasive realm and as medicine continues its trend of replacing invasive treatments with noninvasive treatments such as laser therapy, optometrists and ophthalmologists will increasingly compete with each other for the same types of patients. This likely evolution suggests that only the minority of patients who suffer from exotic eye diseases or require invasive interventions (e.g., cataract surgery, radial keratotomy) will be the sole domain of ophthalmologists. A lot of money should be saved as optometrists are allowed to compete more with ophthalmologists. On services provided both by optometrists and ophthalmologists, the average rate of third-party reimbursement to ophthalmologists is almost 50 percent greater than to optometrists for the same primary care service, i.e., optometrists are paid $41 and ophthalmologists are paid $61 for the same service.[5]

At this point, some readers may wonder if taking so much of eye care out of the sole domain of the ophthalmologist, an M.D., is really healthy. I believe that the answer is "yes" for two reasons. First, a large percentage of the duties undertaken by ophthalmologists, such as routine eye-care testing and procedures, are already within the realm of optometrists, too. Second, exotic diseases of the eye are simply not that common. Ophthalmologists like to defend their supremacy by arguing that optometrists might miss something important, but rare conditions are just that—rare. Besides, optometrists can learn what to look for and can be trusted to refer the rare conditions to an ophthalmologist who knows how to treat them.

Regarding the related insinuation that optometrists simply do not know as much as ophthalmologists, I have from firsthand experience developed considerable skepticism about the scientific base of many things done by physicians. Several years ago—which means things should have improved in the meantime—I served as an expert witness in a hearing involving the scientific validity of optometrists' use of vision training to correct strabismus (misalignment of the eyes). Ophthalmologists had charged that the optometric research on vision training did not prove that vision training worked. They were right; some optometric literature on the subject was scientifically flawed. However, I also evaluated the research that ophthalmologists used to defend their surgical approach to correcting strabismus. The literature on surgical correction was no more scientifically valid than the comparable studies on vision training. Physicians who live in glass houses should not throw stones.

Comparison of Median Annual Net Incomes	
Ophthalmologist (1989)	$205,000
Optometrist (1990)	$68,000
Sources: American Optometric Association, Medical Economics[6]	

---

5. Mort Soroka, "Comparison of Examination Fees and Availability of Routine Vision Care by Optometrists and Ophthalmologists," *Public Health Reports*, vol. 106, no. 4 (July/August 1991).
6. Joel Goldberg, "Opthalmologists' Earnings Shrink," *Medical Economics* (April 12, 1993): 83-96.

Like many medical specialists, ophthalmologists receive extensive *and expensive* medical school training in clinical areas that have nothing to do with diseases of the eye. In fact, they get very little clinical exposure to their specialty until after they graduate from medical school. This inefficient allocation of educational resources again shows that four years of medical school is not a relevant standard for competent patient care. Finally, after anywhere from seven to 10 years of medical education and residency, ophthalmologists begin a private practice where the majority of their work is routine primary care. If society required a comparable background for dentists, they too would be vastly overeducated—and correspondingly more expensive.

Nearly all eye-care needs can be safely provided by optometrists because they are as well educated (perhaps even better educated) *within their specific scope of practice* as ophthalmologists. Like physicians, optometrists begin their advanced degree education after completing (or making significant progress toward) a bachelor's degree. But unlike the ophthalmologists who study to be general medical doctors before specializing in the eye, optometry students spend virtually the entirety of four years in optometry school concentrating on the eye and developing the skills required of their profession. Although they often take twice as much time to master the skills of their profession, ophthalmology students must learn general medicine *and* optometric skills *and* ophthalmologic skills, clearly a daunting task that arguably results in higher costs to recapture the overinvestment.

Jenny

Ray and Susan have noticed that their three-year-old Jenny has crossed eyes. They have been seeing a pediatrician regularly for Jenny's normal childhood problems as well as well-baby care. Jenny's crossed eyes (the condition known as strabismus) have been an ongoing concern for them, but up to this point the pediatrician has wanted to wait until Jenny is older before attempting any therapy. She points out that in some instances the condition is self-correcting. Since Ray and Susan plan to put

Jenny into preschool in the fall, they want to see if something can be done now. They ask for a referral to an eye specialist.

Monopoly model: Jenny's pediatrician refers them to a well-regarded ophthalmologist. After examining Jenny's eyes, the ophthalmologist concludes that her strabismus can be corrected through surgery. He discusses the pros and the cons of the operation. If successful, the problem will be permanently corrected. There is a small chance, however, that as Jenny grows the surgery may have to be redone. There is even a smaller chance, as is true with every surgery, that there may be complications during the operation itself, including death from anesthesia complications. Ray and Susan decide to go ahead with the operation. The surgery turns out to be a success, but the expense puts a strain on the family finances. The total cost of the operation, including physician's fees, hospital, and follow-up is $4,700.00, half of which is covered by Ray's insurance, which he receives through his work.

Competitive model: Jenny's pediatrician recommends she be seen by an optometrist skilled in retraining of the optical muscles. The optometrist describes to Ray and Susan how he can fit Jenny with special glasses and prescribe special eye exercises for her—some of which she must do in the optometrist's office, some at home. He points out that this type of therapy isn't always successful, but the failure rate is about the same for surgery, given its complications and the possibility of having to repeat the operation as Jenny grows older. He also explains that the exercises aren't an instant panacea. They take time and commitment, but they are less stressful on the body than the surgical alternative. Ray and Susan choose to treat Jenny's strabismus using the prescribed plan. The treatment is successful. The cost is $3,400.00, half of which is picked up by the insurance Ray receives through his work.

These comparisons do not diminish the important and unique role of ophthalmologists in eye care. As specialists in reparative eye care involving surgical or aggressive drug intervention, they have proven their worth to many millions of Americans. But the technology of eye care is advancing so fast that many procedures once considered to be "exotic" are now routine. The need for other interventions has been minimized due to new preventive techniques, early diagnosis, and preemptive interventions. Unfortunately, licensing laws have not always recognized these successes nor the fact that optometrists can readily assume more functions once left exclusively to ophthalmologists. Current laws, which were often written in a detailed and limiting manner at the request of medical doctors, need to allow for flexibility as new technology develops. The ability for both ophthalmologists and optometrists to practice in new ways must be dependent on acquiring certification through ongoing education rather than on strict licensing mandates.

Unfortunately, some physician groups, including some organizations of ophthalmologists, are battling these necessary changes. Fortunately, optometrists will not be alone in their battle to assume more responsibility in the field of eye care as an increasing number of allied health professions fight for greater rights to deliver care to a populace in need of a reasonably priced, high-quality alternative.

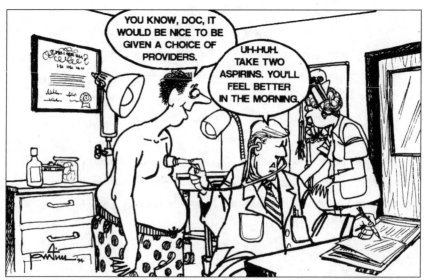

Physical Therapy

> **Physical therapist:** *a person who is licensed to assist in the examination, testing, and treatment of physically disabled or handicapped people through the use of special exercise, application of heat or cold, use of sonar waves, and other techniques.*[7]

Unlike many other allied health providers, physical therapists have already gained a large degree of autonomy in their practice in many states. Traditionally, physical therapists have worked as salaried employees in hospitals and clinics, following doctors' orders for rehabilitating patients. But with the advent of "direct access" in the early 1980s, physical therapists have been permitted the right to practice independently—to evaluate and treat patients without referral from a physician. Today, over 40 states have passed laws acknowledging in various degrees the rights of patients to "directly access" physical therapists.[8]

Like virtually all other nonphysician providers, physical therapists limit themselves to a very specific scope of practice. Nevertheless, they perform a variety of roles, including examining, testing, and treating people who are physically disabled or handicapped. They are also skilled in screening patients with certain physical injuries, a role that was once reserved exclusively for the physician. This responsibility means that while physical therapists can diagnose and treat patients independently from the physician, they must also be knowledgeable and qualified to determine when patients should be referred to a physician.

The practice of physical therapy is noninvasive. It includes massage, manipulation, electric stimulation and therapeutic exercise, cold, heat, and water therapies, and other methods to rehabilitate patients after an illness or injury.[9] Physical therapists do not prescribe drugs for their patients, but they can apply steroid medications to patients' skin. They also cannot order x-rays for patients, but with experience, can interpret about 80 percent of the information presented on x-rays to guide their treatment.[10]

---

7. *Mosby's Medical and Nursing Dictionary*, 2nd edition (St. Louis: C.V. Mosby Company, 1986).
8. Elizabeth Domholdt and Angela Durchholz, "Direct Access Use by Experienced Therapists in States with Direct Access," *Physical Therapy*, vol. 72, no. 8, pp. 569-574.
9. *Mosby's Medical and Nursing Dictionary*, 2nd edition (St. Louis: C.V. Mosby Company, 1986).
10. Linda Karacoloff, Associate Director, Department of Practice, American Physical Therapy Association. Telephone Interview, (May 5, 1993).

> ## Comparison of Mean Annual Incomes
>
> Orthopedist (1991) $248,220
>
> Physical therapist (1993) $42,000
>
> *Sources:* American Physical Therapy Association, Medical Economics[11]

Physical therapists typically earn a Bachelor of Science degree in physical therapy or a special certificate after obtaining a bachelor's degree in a related field.[12] However, more and more physical therapists are earning a master's degree in the field. Physical therapists have chosen to increasingly work in nontraditional environments. In the 1950s, about 80 percent of these therapists worked in a traditional hospital setting. By 1986, however, only 37 percent of them chose to work in a hospital. Most physical therapists now work in home health care agencies, rehabilitation centers, extended-care facilities, school programs, and academic institutions. The number of therapists in private practice is expected to be much larger today than the 18 percent reported in 1986.[13]

Even though many states give physical therapists the right to at least some independent practice, the therapists are not always able to do so. The most significant roadblock to "direct access" is the third-party practice of requiring patients to see a doctor before reimbursing for physical therapy treatments. When this occurs in states that have legalized direct access, physical therapists are effectively forced to operate under physician control again, essentially defeating the direct-access concept. (Again, monopoly works in subtle ways.) In fact, almost one-third of physical therapists responding to a 1989 survey stated that they had problems obtaining reimbursement for direct-access practice.[14]

Physical therapists, like other allied health professionals, face real problems in their efforts to work as independent professionals *with* doctors rather than *for* doctors. When direct access is implemented and has the full cooperation of

11. Arthur Owens, "What's the Recession Done to Your Buying Power?" *Medical Economics* (Sept 7, 1992): 197.
12. *Mosby's Medical and Nursing Dictionary*, 2nd edition (St. Louis: C.V. Mosby Company, 1986).
13. Charles Magistro, "Clinical Decision Making in Physical Therapy: A Practitioner's Perspective," *Physical Therapy*, vol. 69, no. 7 (July 1989): 525-533.
14. Domholdt and Durchholz, pp. 569-574.

insurance companies, the patient's total cost of care is reduced because the unnecessary middleman—the physician—is cut out of the loop. Thus, complete independence hinges not only on rewriting state medical practice acts, but on redesigning insurance reimbursement programs to recognize physical therapists and other qualified allied health practitioners as equal partners to physicians in the delivery of health care.

Winfred

At 51, Winfred feels he has a few more years left before turning over his family-owned, family-operated hog farm to his sons. He still works 10- to 12-hour days, and though he realizes he's slowing down, he claims he can still keep up with "the youngsters," as he calls his sons. But one afternoon while cleaning out the hog pens, he feels a muscle pull in his back. He completes the job with only a slight twinge of pain. The next morning Winfred wakes up and feels very intense pain in his lower back as he tries to get out of bed. He flops back on the mattress and cries for his wife, Frances. By the afternoon, Winfred can move slightly, and with a lot of assistance from his wife, he walks slowly to the car.

Monopoly model: *Winfred's wife, Frances, takes him to the local hospital where he is seen in the emergency room. A doctor examines him and determines that he has a severely pulled muscle. He prescribes anti-inflammatory medications, pain medications, and physical therapy treatments. The cost is $150 for the hospital visit and $55 for the medications, for a total cost of $205.*

Competitive model: *Frances takes Winfred to the town's physical therapist who shares a clinic with the local nurse practitioner. The physical therapist determines that Winfred has a pulled muscle and that there is no nerve damage. She starts Winfred on a physical therapy regimen and consults with the nurse practitioner who orders medications for inflammation and pain. The cost of the initial clinic visit is $40, and the medications are $35, for a total cost of $75.*

Pharmacist

Pharmacist: a specialist in formulating and dispensing medications.[15]

The pharmacy profession offers some particularly exciting possibilities. Today, pharmacists in most states spend the majority of their time filling prescriptions written by physicians. They receive the prescriptions from physicians, fill the order, and dispense the medicine. About 20 percent of their time is devoted to patient education and counseling.[16] Historically, pharmacists have not always held so limited a role. Throughout the middle ages and even up until the end of the nineteenth century, particularly in Europe, pharmacists were considered an equal choice in the health care provider spectrum, along with physicians, midwives, and barber-surgeons. Each had a role to fill, and none was beholden to the other.

In Europe as well as many other parts of the world today, especially where the supply of physicians is limited, pharmacists continue to play a major role in diagnosing and treating minor illnesses. They do not set bones, deliver babies, or perform surgeries, but they do prescribe medicines—one of the roles that the American physician has reserved solely for himself in the twentieth century. This has led to one of the great ironies of our medical system: pharmacists on the whole are much more extensively schooled in pharmacology (the study of drugs and their appropriate uses) than most of the physicians from whom they receive their orders. Pharmacists, for instance, must take five years of clinical training in order to obtain a Doctor of Pharmacology (Pharm.D.) degree; almost all of these five years is devoted to the study of medicines and their effects on the body. Medical students, on the other hand, often take as little as three classes in pharmacology before earning their M.D. degrees and receiving the unquestioned right to prescribe drugs.

Today's pharmacist is certainly capable of diagnosing many common ailments using computerized diagnostic tools, commercially available tests, and laboratory services. More importantly, however, the pharmacist's role can and should

---

15. *Mosby's Medical and Nursing Dictionary*, 2nd edition (St. Louis: C.V. Mosby Company, 1986).
16. Heidi M. Anderson-Harper, et. al., "Pharmacists' Predisposition to Communicate, Desire to Counsel and Job Satisfaction," *American Journal of Pharmaceutical Education*, vol. 56 (Fall 1992): 252-258.

be to determine the appropriate drug (or no drug, if the protocols so suggest) based on diagnoses provided by other independent practitioners such as physicians, nurse practitioners, nurse midwives, and psychologists (who at present cannot prescribe).

Lucy

Lucy is 14 and loves to swim. One day after a visit to the public pool, she develops raised, red, itchy patches on her skin. She shows them to her mother, who has never seen anything like them before. The family health insurance does not cover visits to the doctor, so Lucy's mother doesn't know whether she should seek medical treatment or simply hope that the rash will go away.

Monopoly model: Three days after the rash started to develop, Lucy's mom finally decides to make an appointment for Lucy to see a doctor. By this time, Lucy's unconscious itching of the rash has made the condition worse. Once in the office, the doctor examines the rash, makes a diagnosis, and prescribes a steroid-based cream. Lucy's mom fills the prescription at her local pharmacy. The doctor's visit costs $35, and the cream is an additional $15; the total cost is $50.

Competitive model: The day after the rash appears, Lucy's mom decides to take Lucy to the local pharmacy. A few minutes after arriving, a pharmacist examines the rash and asks Lucy questions about her health history. The pharmacist then enters the information into a computer and accesses the software package that confirms the initial diagnosis. He determines the adequate treatment based on the information on the computer and prescribes a steroid-based cream. The pharmacist charges a $10 consultation fee and $15 for the cream; the total cost is $25.

While many physicians would like to protect their monopoly by claiming that healing is an art, the truth is that many of the diagnostic and healing processes today can be reduced to protocols—guidelines on how to narrow down the possibilities to the most likely diagnosis. When a patient's symptoms are entered into a database, a computerized analysis can isolate the probable problem, from which a treatment (or alternative treatments) can be determined based on past cases of dealing with those symptoms. While these computerized methods of determining and choosing a treatment for an illness work well in a doctor's office, they can be utilized just as easily by a trained pharmacist. (Many physicians complain about the arrival of "cookbook medicine," but computer-based protocols are effectively little more than the application of modern technology—the computer—and decision science to the doctor's traditional art of differential diagnosis. Perhaps some part of the doctors' dislike for protocols is related to the fact that computer-assisted diagnosis is so readily accessible to nonphysician providers.)

If a patient with flu-like symptoms goes to a drug store instead of a doctor's office (or even a nurse practitioner's office—isn't free market competition wonderful?), the pharmacist could ask the patient questions to determine the severity of the problem and to identify the patient's medical history. The pharmacist could then consult the computer to check the patient's record and access another file that helps determine the diagnosis. During the visit, the pharmacist could also collect a sputum specimen to identify the offending bacteria or take a throat culture to test for strep throat. (Neither of these procedures requires medical school training. In fact, patients are allowed to test themselves in some modern countries where people are healthier than we Americans.) Following the consultation, the pharmacist could then prescribe the appropriate antibiotic or other medication. If the patient has an underlying respiratory problem, e.g., asthma or emphysema, then the pharmacist would refer the patient to a physician or other qualified nonphysician provider. The pharmacist would be qualified to diagnose and prescribe only upon completion of specific certification.

Allowing diagnostic tools and the power of writing prescriptions to be handed over to pharmacists, if even on a limited basis, would naturally be a scary thing for many physicians—as well as some consumers. Doctors' warnings about the "dangers" of an "untrained" pharmacist with a computer might have a strong emotional appeal. But we must keep in mind that some commentators argue that as many as one-third of all physician diagnoses and treatments may be either incorrect, ineffective, or damaging to the patient.[17] Of course, like any independent health care practitioner, a pharmacist must always be responsible for referring any patient whose condition is beyond his or her scope of practice to a more appropriate provider, such as a physician, nurse practitioner, physical therapist, nurse midwife, dentist, or psychologist.

While allowing pharmacists to diagnose and prescribe may sound futuristic and even unrealistic, a model of this type of expanded role already exists. On May 1, 1986, Florida passed the Pharmacist Self-Care Consultant Law, which gives community pharmacists independent authority to prescribe specific medications used to treat mild, self-limiting conditions. The list of prescription medications includes certain antihistamines and decongestants; hemorrhoid aids; oral, otic (ear), and urinary analgesics; anti-nausea preparations; anti-inflammatory agents; and fluorides. In California, Washington, and Mississippi, pharmacists also have been allowed to prescribe certain drugs according to previously determined physician protocols.[18]

Both pharmacists and consumers are beginning to see the benefits of the Florida experiment. One pharmacist has stated that the law "acknowledges the pharmacist's education and ability to handle minor medical problems." Another pharmacist notes that patients are now able "to get treatment quicker, faster, and at less expense for a minor ailment." Overall, many pharmacists view the new system as cost-effective for consumers.[19]

---

17. For related discussion, see C. Phelps, "The Methodological Foundations of the Appropriateness of Medical Care." *New England Journal of Medicine* 329: 17 (October 21, 1993): pp. 1241-1245.
18. For further discussion, see H. Eng, "Developments in Pharmacy Practice," *Journal of Clinical Pharmacy and Therapeutics* (December 1987): 237-242; and I. Rosendahl, "Pharmacist Prescribing is Off to a Cautious Start," *Drug Topics* (February 16, 1987): 54-64.
19. I. Rosendahl, p. 56.

Connie

Connie, 33, lives in a small town and works as an accountant. She is also the mother of two young boys. Recently, her husband sustained injuries on his construction job and is not able to work. This added pressure, plus a conflict with her supervisor, has rekindled a feeling of depression that has plagued her off and on throughout her life. She has been seeing a local psychologist periodically and feels she has benefited from his help. However, the current strain is just too much, and now she thinks she needs some sort of medication.

Monopoly model: The psychologist explains to Connie that he cannot order a medication for her and suggests a psychiatrist (an allopathically trained M.D.) in a town 20 miles away. Unfortunately, the psychiatrist is outside the preferred provider network of Connie's medical insurance. Despite the added financial pressure of her husband being out of work, Connie reasons that she will only need to visit the psychiatrist once. She makes an appointment. The psychiatrist uses their entire 50-minute consultation to take her psychological history, information that her own psychologist already knows. At the end of the session, he prescribes a well-known medication. The charge for Connie's visit is $125 for the consultation, plus $75 for one month's supply of pills, for a total cost of $200.

Competitive model: Connie's psychologist explains that he cannot prescribe a medication for her, but he can supply necessary information and make a recommendation to the local pharmacist who is certified to write prescriptions following certain protocols. The psychologist and the pharmacist agree that while a well-known medication may be advisable, recent studies have indicated that it can have adverse side effects and may be addictive. Instead, the pharmacist chooses a proven generic medication (one where the patent no longer applies), which may not act as quickly but which has a history of less dangerous side effects. The cost to Connie is the 20 percent co-pay on a $75 office visit with the psychologist, or $15, plus $16 for a month's supply of pills and a $5 prescribing fee to the pharmacist. Her total out-of-pocket cost is $36.

As with other nonphysician providers who have historically been beholden to doctors' orders, many pharmacists will need additional training in order to prescribe medications. This training could be acquired through a series of certificate programs for pharmacists already established in practice. Pharmacy students could also train for expanded responsibilities in pharmacy school. Already, many of these schools are expanding their curriculum by adding new courses or replacing less essential courses with ones that are more clinically oriented.

Comparison of Income

Clinical pharmacist* (1992 mean) $49,150

Family practice physician (1991 median) $101,160

*A clinical pharmacist educates patients in the hospital about their
medications and is consulted frequently by physicians.
Sources: American Society of Hospital Pharmacists, Medical Economics[20]

As with other nonphysician providers, pharmacists must be free to choose whether to take on the added responsibility of writing prescriptions. Here again, individual certification should be as important as basic education and general licensure. Beginning in pharmacy school, a pharmacist could "move up the career ladder" according to his or her own interests and timetable. A pharmaceutical education *plus* a license would admit the pharmacist to traditional practice, that is, filling doctors' prescriptions and providing patient education. A pharmaceutical education *plus* a license *plus* certification for writing prescriptions would allow the pharmacist to make diagnoses and prescribe medicines for certain conditions. A student who chooses not to pursue a course leading to expanded practice in pharmacy school could opt to do so later through accredited certification courses.

While the small steps made in Florida, California, Washington, and Mississippi provide a good start, a more sweeping effort needs to be made in order for pharmacists to take on greater responsibilities in diagnosing minor illnesses and prescribing appropriate medications. There is no longer a need to funnel all health care through the physician, adding an unnecessary and expensive

---

20. Arthur Owens, "What's the Recession Done to Your Buying Power?" *Medical Economics*
(Sept 7, 1992): 197.

middleman to what should be a simple and relatively inexpensive process. The obligatory visit to the physician just to get a prescription will be reduced if patients can go straight to a pharmacist instead for basic problems. Expanding pharmacists' authority to match their training will be just one more step toward creating a more accessible and less costly health care system for all citizens.

As an endnote to this discussion, I must admit to some personal frustration with the number of pharmacists who have told me that they do not want to have prescribing authority even though they will also tell me that they truly believe they could prescribe much more appropriately than physicians. Commonly, the first explanation for this reluctance is fear of professional liability, but a little more conversation usually gets around to what I suspect is the real reason: fear that physicians will turn to dispensing drugs in their offices if pharmacists start prescribing drugs in their pharmacies. Some turnabout is fair play, but I think that many consumers would prefer to have their medication prescribed by a pharmacist following physical assessment by a doctor or qualified nonphysician—once they understand the relative differences in prescribing skills. I also expect that insurance companies will ultimately favor prescribing by qualified pharmacists because pharmacists would be less likely than doctors to order an unnecessary drug if the compensation for dispensing were separated from the price of the drug. Pharmacists' fears of physicians' control over their incomes may delay the time when consumers will benefit from prescribing pharmacists, but competition is a powerful force once unleashed. Stay tuned for further details.

Jamie

Jamie, 30, is a paralegal in a large office that currently has several people at home with strep throat. On Friday, Jamie discovers that his throat is increasingly sore and that it hurts to talk. By the end of the day, he is extremely fatigued and feels chilled. When he gets home, he takes his temperature and discovers that it's 102° F. He then examines his throat with a flashlight and discovers white patches on his tonsils.

Monopoly model: *Jamie realizes that his doctor will not be available until Monday. He contemplates going to the emergency room at the nearby hospital but decides instead to wait to see his doctor. He spends the weekend in bed, missing a social engagement that had been planned for weeks. On Monday, he calls in sick, then phones his doctor's office for an appointment. The receptionist tells him that the doctor can see him at four o'clock. Jamie knows from experience that he will be among others who have had to make emergency appointments, and that he will have to wait. At 4:45 p.m., Jamie finally is able to see his physician. The doctor examines Jamie, performs a throat culture, confirms a strep infection, and prescribes an antibiotic. The visit with the doctor is $35, the cost of the throat culture $17, and the price of the antibiotic $30, for a total cost of $82, none of which is covered by Jamie's insurance.*

Competitive model: *Jamie visits the local pharmacy that Friday evening. The pharmacist swabs his throat with a quick test strip and asks Jamie about his health history. He updates Jamie's patient record on his computer, examines the test strip, and consults the computerized diagnostic base to confirm his preliminary diagnosis and recommended treatment. The computer file also recommends when a patient should see another health professional, depending on the presence of certain symptoms. The pharmacist then prescribes an antibiotic, instructs Jamie on how to deal with the illness, and tells him to take it easy for awhile. Jamie still misses his social engagement, but he feels much better by Monday morning. The total cost of the visit is $15 for the pharmacist's consulting fee, $5 for the test strip, and $30 for the antibiotic, for a total of $50. Jamie is able to return to work on Monday.*

Chapter Eight

Competitive Options in Allied Health

Nurse practitioners, certified nurse midwives, dentists, pharmacists, and physical therapists have made the greatest advances toward creation of a more competitive medical marketplace—albeit to varying degrees—but a few allied health professionals are also poised to challenge the medical monopoly. This chapter presents these additional options and shows how consumers would be better off if they were free to choose from an expanded menu of qualified providers.

Respiratory Therapist

> **Respiratory Therapist:** *a person who, under the supervision of a physician, administers oxygen and other gases and provides assistance to patients with breathing difficulties. A respiratory therapist who has successfully completed the examination of the National Board for Respiratory Care (NBRC) is designated as a registered respiratory therapist.*[1]

---

1. *Mosby's Medical and Nursing Dictionary,* 2nd edition (St. Louis: C.V. Mosby Company, 1986).

Respiratory therapists (RTs) are yet another nonphysician provider group capable of independent practice within their defined scope of practice. Through direct access and mandated reimbursement, they could be available to offer many important health services traditionally administered only by or through physicians. Operating under standardized protocols, respiratory therapists are capable of offering basic pulmonary evaluations, diagnoses, and treatments for such medical problems as asthma, pulmonary emphysema, chronic bronchitis, cystic fibrosis, and black lung disease. They are also trained to prescribe such medications as bronchodilators, mucolytics, and atropine.

Operated by independent therapists with advanced training and certification, respiratory therapy clinics could offer allergy and asthma sufferers an alternative to the traditional (and expensive) physician's office or clinic—offering maintenance services such as management of chronic emphysema and emergency treatment at a dramatic cost savings compared to hospital emergency rooms. In these clinics, qualified respiratory therapists could diagnose the condition, administer inhaled medications and therapy, and provide patient education.

Since many patients with a new respiratory disease might prefer the more diagnostically oriented physician or nurse practitioner, the specialized role of independent respiratory therapists could be maintenance care for patients with chronic respiratory diseases. Independent therapists could provide respiratory care to patients in their homes, including management of patients on ventilators (mechanical devices that assist breathing). Indeed, qualified respiratory therapists could provide a lower-cost, comparable quality alternative to home health services that are currently dependent upon a physician as the "middle man" for respiratory treatments (see "Home Health Care Providers" later in this chapter). The independent respiratory therapists could also be qualified to provide preventive care in nursing homes and other long-term care centers. For example, they could assess the pneumonia risk of bedridden institutionalized patients and intervene before the patients' conditions warranted hospitalization.

Many respiratory therapists function with some autonomy in hospitals today. Operating under protocol systems that establish decision-making guidelines, respiratory therapists determine patient treatment programs. In many systems, they can order indicated tests, though they cannot order invasive procedures. These treatment plans are then reviewed daily by designated peers to ensure appropriate care was administered. The success of such programs bolsters arguments advanced by many respiratory therapists—they are capable of operating more independently outside the hospital and developing their own protocols for independent practice.

Just as we saw in other nonphysician health professions, there are progressive levels of education and certification in the training of respiratory therapists. Students wishing to become respiratory therapy technicians can be trained and certified within 12 months, but certification as a Registered Respiratory Therapist (RRT) only occurs after a 24-month training program and passing national exams. RRTs who wish to further their education may earn a Bachelor's Degree in Respiratory Therapy (BSRRT) after a four-year program. Today, respiratory therapists may continue their education to the master's and doctorate levels, but the latter only in areas such as public health or health administration. The accelerated development of advanced clinical degrees in respiratory therapy should probably be an important part of overall efforts to qualify graduate-trained respiratory therapists for independent practice.

Comparison of Net Income, 1990	
Respiratory Therapist (Mean)	$30,264
Family Practice Physician (Median)	$98,290
Source: American Association for Respiratory Care, Medical Economics[2]	

2. Arthur Owens, "Doctors Struggle to Stay Ahead of Inflation," *Medical Economics* (September 2, 1991).

Louise

Louise is a 69-year-old woman with chronic emphysema. She has smoked about two packs a day for most of her adult years and only quit smoking four years ago. She has noticed that it is becoming increasingly difficult to work in her yard without becoming short of breath, and she is coughing more heavily in the mornings upon awakening.

Monopoly model: Louise makes an appointment to see her pulmonologist (a specialized M.D.) the following week. During the physician visit, she describes her symptoms and reviews her medications. He checks her oxygenation via an ear oximetry test and takes a blood sample to monitor her medication levels. He then monitors her tolerance to some simple exercise and suggests some modifications to her daily routine. At the end of the visit, he adjusts her medication dose and charges her $50 for the visit.

Competitive model: Louise visits a local respiratory center located in the shopping mall near her home. She describes her symptoms to the certified respiratory therapist and shows her the type of pills she is currently taking. The respiratory therapist takes a blood sample to monitor the patient's blood levels of theophylline, a medication used to dilate the airways and make breathing easier. The respiratory therapist adjusts the dosage of the theophylline pills following protocol developed by a group of respiratory therapists and pulmonologists. Before prescribing an exercise program, the respiratory therapist uses a simple test to measure Louise's oxygenation while at rest and during a light exercise program to determine her tolerance and need for oxygen supplementation. After Louise discusses the findings and recommendations with the therapist, she then leaves the respiratory center with an adjusted dose of her medication and a new exercise program. The cost for the visit is $35.

The licensure of respiratory therapists varies from state to state. Also, some conflicts exist between respiratory therapists and other nonphysician providers. For example, should registered nurses be allowed to administer oxygen in nursing homes, or should this task be left only to respiratory therapists? However, all the conflicts can be resolved as part of coordinated efforts to make sure that RRTs with advanced training, like other qualified nonphysician providers, are recognized for their ability to provide specific health care free from physician control.

Occupational Therapy

Like their counterparts in physical therapy and respiratory therapy, occupational therapists can offer preventive services that save the employer substantial health care expenses in the long term. For example, prolonged computer use is increasingly linked to a new group of medical problems called Cumulative Trauma Disorders, or overuse injuries that strain the nerves involved in work-related tasks. Occupational therapists can work with people at risk to modify their jobs, thus preventing the worn-out, inflamed tendons that are becoming increasingly common in computer workers. With a preventive outlay of $300 to $1,000 for occupational therapy intervention, the employer is spared thousands of dollars in surgery and worker's compensation claims, and the employee is spared life-long pain, career-limiting injury, and possible loss of income.

Occupational therapists are also very skilled at teaching a patient how to cope with basic activities of daily living after he or she has experienced an injury or illness. They are especially useful in assisting with problems related to neurologically oriented disorders such as strokes. Occupational therapists have special training in psychology and are also equipped to teach stress management and prevention skills. The profession's goal is to help people become functional in their environments through the use of healthy coping strategies. Unfortunately, most people are unaware of the full range of occupational therapists' skills. For example, occupational therapists can work to restore range of motion to hands that have recently been immobilized with splints, but many patients experience long-term problems because they never receive this important service.

Carl

Carl is a nine-year-old boy who has a history of allergies. One Saturday he is visiting relatives at their farm. Suddenly, he begins to cough and wheeze. His eyes swell shut. His parents recognize this as a full-blown asthma attack, probably due to the animals and grasses. Carl then breathes through his inhaler, which enables him to breathe a little easier. While the family has learned to cope with these attacks, this one appears to be more serious than any he has had before. They realize Carl needs immediate medical attention. Fortunately, there is a medium-sized town less than half an hour away.

Monopoly model: Carl's mother takes him to the town's hospital for treatment. He receives a physical assessment by the emergency room doctor, an ear oximetry test, blood tests, chest x-ray, adrenaline, and other medications. His total bill for the treatment is $530, which includes the use of the emergency room ($125), physician visit ($125), and medications and tests ($280).

Competitive model: After calling ahead, Carl's mother decides to take him to a health center that is owned and operated by nurse practitioners and respiratory therapists. The center is open on Saturday for the convenience of its working and school-aged patients. A respiratory therapist performs a physical assessment, administers appropriate tests, and delivers the medications via an aerosol and by mouth. The total bill is $180, which includes the clinic visit and the medications and tests.

In some states, occupational therapists can practice independently, that is, patients can refer themselves to OT without a physician's prescription. Once again, however, occupational therapists' ability to practice independently is often hindered because many insurance companies require that all patient visits must be authorized by a physician before reimbursement is approved.

Thus, even in states that allow independent practice, patients can be forced to see physicians before purchasing occupational therapy services if the service is to be paid by the third party. This arrangement virtually negates the benefit of independent practice.

Edith

Edith is a 50-year-old female who has worked for the past few years as a data entry clerk at the local university hospital. Lately, she's noticed increasing pain and weakness in her wrists and hands when working at the keyboard. On a few occasions, the pain has even radiated up her forearm toward her shoulder.

Monopoly model: *Edith sees her family physician, who recommends surgery for carpal tunnel syndrome. The total cost for the day surgery, which includes surgeon's fees, is $4,000.*

Competitive model: *When Edith initially starts her job as data entry clerk, she spends several hours with one of the hospital's occupational therapists, who helps alter the layout of the data entry position at her desk and teaches Edith some exercises designed to prevent carpal tunnel injury. Years later, Edith is working comfortably, utilizing the information she learned from the occupational therapist. The total cost of the evaluation and intervention by the occupational therapist was $300.*

Unfortunately, this problem prevails in most states because so many insurance companies are national organizations with rules that transcend state borders. Many occupational therapists are still tied to the physician, and the public is denied the opportunity to purchase their services directly. Even if all states were to recognize occupational therapists' qualifications for independent practice, the field of occupational therapy would be a greater asset to American health if the insurance restrictions were also removed and if the public were better educated about their capabilities.

Audiologists

> *Audiologist:* a professional dedicated to the field of hearing, especially impaired hearing that cannot be corrected by medical means.[3]

The relationship between audiologists and physicians is remarkably similar to the relationship between optometrists and ophthalmologists, with one large difference: while optometrists practice with a relatively advanced degree of independence, only a few states allow professional autonomy to audiologists. And yet, like optometrists, audiologists are fully qualified to perform many functions generally reserved to the control of physicians. In most states, an individual with a hearing problem must first visit a physician to rule out surgery or medical intervention before being fitted for a hearing aid. That's like requiring a child who has trouble seeing the classroom blackboard to visit a pediatrician or an ophthalmologist before receiving glasses, or requiring a senior citizen with a toothache to see a doctor before being sent to a dentist.

Most individuals with hearing loss will never need medical intervention, but professional practice acts still force them to see a physician. However, audiologists today are capable of performing the initial screening to determine the patient's condition and the necessity of physician referral. If indicated, they can then proceed to fit the patients with hearing aids. These professionals are very experienced in the diagnosis and dispensing of hearing aids, which is the bulk of their private practice.

Audiologists are trained to perform many auditory diagnostic tests without physician supervision, including screening and managing patients who are experiencing dizziness or ringing in the ears. They are also well equipped to diagnose communication disorders in children. Pediatricians are not generally well trained in audiology and often must refer their young patients to audiologists for these special screenings. Parents could save a lot of money if they knew they could take their symptomatic child directly to an audiologist.

---

3. *Mosby's Medical and Nursing Dictionary*, 2nd edition (St. Louis: C.V. Mosby Company, 1986).

Determining the degree of disability involving hearing loss and the appropriate workers' compensation is an expanding area of need that can be met by independent audiologists. Traditionally, the evaluation of hearing loss has been exclusively in the hands of doctors, but audiologists have the most specific training in this area. In addition, industrial hearing conservation is becoming an important branch of occupational health; audiologists are well-suited to supervise or direct the related preventive programs. The expanded use of independent audiologists in such clinical roles should be welcomed by the many physicians who complain that worksite regulations have forced them to shift from patient care to paper shuffling. Audiologists can relieve physicians of the administrative burden and provide perfectly acceptable care in special areas like industrial medicine. Needless to say, a little competition between audiologists and doctors ought to give employers a chance to reduce the overall costs of health care for their employees.

Comparison of Median Annual Incomes

Family Practice (1991) $101,160

Audiologist (1992) $ 35,782

Source: American Speech-Language-Hearing Association,
Medical Economics[4]

The minimum requirement for audiologists is a masters degree, one year of clinical experience, and passing a national exam. Many students continue to pursue doctoral degrees in audiology. Audiologists are licensed by most, but not all, states. However, states that do not license audiologists often allow the distinction between audiologists and hearing aid dealers (who do not have professional, graduate training) to remain blurred—a clear disservice to the consumer.

---

4. Arthur Owens, "What's the Recession Done to Your Buying Power?" *Medical Economics* (September 7, 1992): 197.

Li

At age 72, Li is increasingly frustrated with his inability to hear. His wife has been encouraging him to have a hearing evaluation for over a year now, but he has stubbornly resisted. Finally, at a Thanksgiving party, when Li realizes he can't hear his grandchildren clearly, he decides to seek treatment.

Monopoly model: *Li schedules an appointment with an ear, nose, and throat (ENT) doctor to have his hearing checked. The doctor examines Li's ears, performs the necessary hearing tests, and refers Li to an audiologist to be fitted with a hearing aid. The cost of the physician visit is $56. The visit with the audiologist and the exam is an additional $100; the hearing aids are $750. The total cost to the patient for all health care services is $906.*

Competitive model: *Li makes an appointment directly with an audiologist, who examines his ears and tests his hearing. The audiologist checks first for disease or any other physiological disorder that would require physician intervention. Satisfied that Li's problem is a simple form of hearing loss due to his advancing years, the audiologist fits Li with two hearing aids. The cost of the initial visit and exam is $100, and the hearing aids are $750. The total cost to the patient is $850.*

Not surprisingly—given what we have already seen in doctors' subtle control over health insurance—one of the most significant problems that audiologists face in achieving independent status is obtaining direct reimbursement from third-party payers. In almost all cases, third-party reimbursement is tied to physician referral. This forced linkage to a physician undermines the ability of audiologists to diagnose problems because it effectively gives a physician the final say. Strangely enough, Medicare goes halfway on this issue, reimbursing audiologists only for exams on patients who do not need hearing aids. Thus, physicians are the only providers reimbursed by Medicare for testing patients who need hearing aids.[5] (Does this make sense to anyone?) In many

---

5. Steve White, director of Health Care Financing at the American Speech-Language-Hearing Association. Personal interview (March 31, 1993).

cases, audiologists employed by physicians do the clinical work anyway, allowing physicians to take a cut of the Medicare payment simply by processing the paperwork. Not only does this systemic flaw keep audiologists under the thumb of physicians, but it sets Medicare reimbursement rates at the level of physicians' fees rather than the more modest charges of the nonphysician providers.

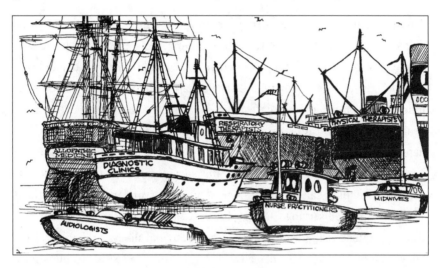

Compared to optometry and dentistry, audiology is a relatively new nonphysician provider specialty. Yet it has made great progress in the recent past. For example, audiologists' role in public health is well known to any parent taking his or her child to a pre-kindergarten screening. But one of the problems with our health care system is the sharp division between public health (which deals with health at the level of populations) and medical care for individual patients. While nonphysicians are deemed "adequate" to act as key personnel in the realm of public health, only the physician is generally regarded as an acceptable authority in the realm of individual health. It is logical, then, for audiologists to be freed to translate the skills they have developed in public health and in working for physicians into their own independent practice. Like optometrists, audiologists are qualified to take over more of the physicians' responsibility in diagnosing and treating common problems within their scope of practice. Not only will this mean the availability of a competing medical service, but it will also free up physicians' valuable time for more complicated medical challenges.

Dental Hygienist

> **Dental hygienist:** *a person with special training to provide dental services under the supervision of a dentist. Services supplied by a dental hygienist include dental prophylaxis, radiography, application of medications, and provision of dental education at chairside and in the community.*[6]

Although dental hygiene lies firmly within the realm of dentistry rather than medicine, I include it here for two reasons. First, registered dental hygienists, like many other allied health practitioners, are capable of being the initial contact for individuals entering into the health care system, and they can do so as independent providers in several states. Notice I say "individuals entering the health care system" rather than "patients needing medical assistance" because dentists, far more than physicians, have been very successful in promoting preventive or "wellness" care. Part of this success is due to the nature of the specialty. Dentists can advocate regular checkups and prevention without seeming to be self-serving. Dental disease can be discovered and controlled through regular visits to the dentist, while potential illness to the rest of the body cannot be so easily detected during routine physical examinations. Furthermore, dentists get paid for preventive prophylaxis work (teeth cleaning). The best the physicians can do is recommend a healthy diet, regular exercise, stress avoidance, adequate sleep, moderate alcohol consumption, and no smoking—none of which earns them a dime.

The second reason for including dental hygienists is that the field of dentistry is itself a perfect example of how well the health system can work when qualified nonphysician providers are allowed to be captains of their own ships. As previously noted, dentistry evolved into a profession separate from medicine before physicians established their monopoly over diagnosis and treatment. We take this separation for granted; in fact, it seems perfectly logical to us that dentists are totally independent of physician control. The mouth is a clinically distinct part of the body with its own anatomy and physiology. That the mouth should have its own doctor makes sense.

---

6. *Mosby's Medical and Nursing Dictionary*, 2nd edition (St. Louis: C.V. Mosby Company, 1986).

Julio

Twelve-year-old Julio has gone without dental care for most of his life. Preventive dental care is simply too expensive for his migrant worker parents who must support a large extended family. As a result, he has already lost one tooth to dental decay and is currently experiencing pain in another tooth.

Monopoly model: Julio's father must miss a day of work to drive his son 100 miles to find a dentist willing to treat patients at a substantial discount. Julio receives a dental prophylaxis (cleaning) and has a filling placed in one tooth. In addition, a dental hygienist gives him instructions on proper tooth care. The cost to Julio's father is $70, a substantial discount from the normal dentist's fee of $140. But he also loses about $80 in what he'd earn in the fields for a day's wages.

Competitive model: Julio visits a nearby health clinic set up to treat patients from low-income families and operated by non-physician providers. He sees a dental hygienist, who immediately ascertains that Julio has a cavity that needs filling. The dental hygienist cleans Julio's teeth and instructs him in the proper methods of dental health, including correct eating habits, proper brushing habits, and flossing. The next day, a dentist who visits the clinic on a regular basis fills the cavity. Afterwards, the dental hygienist strongly encourages Julio and his family to visit the clinic once a year for routine checkups and cleanings. The cost of the service is $35 for the checkup and cleaning, plus $30 for the filling, for a total of $65. Julio's father does not lose any wages.

Dentistry has remained separate from traditional medicine, maintaining its own schools and clearly defining its scope of practice. Unlike other medical specialists, future dentists are not required to take a four-year course of general medical study before pursuing their specialty; the dental school curriculum is efficiently designed to match instruction to actual practice needs. Nor are patients required to get a physician referral before going to a dentist. For these reasons, dentistry has been an attractive profession to those wishing to pursue a career in medicine but not wanting to become physicians. Dentistry has also been less influenced by the third-party payer system. Most patients still pay substantial portions of their dental bills. Thanks to the stronger financial relationship between patient and dentist, to the efficiency of dental education, and to the absence of institutional care—most dentists practice in small offices and clinics rather than in hospitals—dentistry has remained more responsive to individual health care needs than traditional allopathic medicine. The increased independence of the registered dental hygienist has beneficially added a competitive element within dentistry, keeping dentists responsive because patients have a choice.

Today, well-trained dental hygienists are clinically qualified to provide their specialized services in their own offices. A dentist does not need to tell them what to do, and registered dental hygienists know well what they cannot do and must refer to a dentist. In addition, the hygienist offers a much less threatening point of entry for individuals who know they need dental care but fear going to the dentist. (One study showed that 28 percent of the respondents were more likely to seek care from a practice without a dentist.[7]) In addition, the Julio scenario shows how dental hygiene can be incorporated into a comprehensive health clinic (or "wellness center") operated by nonphysician providers, offering preventive dental care and early screening as part of regular health care. In this scenario, a dentist is needed only to fill cavities, perform oral surgery, and provide the various other restorative and reconstructive services that reflect the advanced training of a doctor. Because an independent hygienist does not have the high overhead and administrative costs related to dental surgery, his or her preventive and diagnostic services can cost less than the same services provided by a dentist (or even the same services provided by a hygienist in a dentist's office). In addition to this cost advantage for basic services, a comprehensive clinic with basic dental services can mean that families like Julio's will be more likely to get routine, preventive dental care.

---

7. "Final Report Health Manpower Pilot Project," *American Dental Hygienists' Association*, (January 1987-December 1989): 14.

Rose

Rose is 88 and lives in a nursing home. Usually, the nursing home requires that all its residents see a dentist once a year and it has assumed the cost of transporting them to a nearby clinic. But the expense of these visits has become prohibitive for some residents, and the logistics of the transportation has never been easy. The nursing home is therefore considering dropping the annual dental visit program.

Monopoly model: *The nursing home decides to change the annual dental visit from a requirement to a recommendation, changing the policy from making the arrangements to assisting in making the arrangements, as requested by the resident or resident's family.*

Competitive model: *The nursing home management contracts with a private dental health service operated by dental hygienists. Once a year for all residents, and once every six months for some residents (according to a prearranged agreement with the resident or resident's family), the dental health service sends a van and team of dental hygienists to the nursing home.*

Dental hygienists also provide a good model for qualified nonphysician providers' potential contributions to public health. Sadly, one of the consequences of the physician monopoly has been the separation of medical care from public health. Some medical theorists, most notably Rick J. Carlson in *The End of Medicine*, argue very convincingly that medicine has been given far too much emphasis and public health too little, despite the fact that public health has done far more to prolong human life and alleviate human suffering than medical intervention.[8] *The field of health economics has abundant evidence that the cost-benefit ratio is much higher for a dollar spent on public health than for a dollar spent on individual medical care.*

---

8. Rick J. Carlson, *The End of Medicine* (New York: John Wiley & Sons, 1975).

Dentistry as a profession has proven itself a champion of preventive care and patient education, but poor oral health is still one of the most serious problems for our nation's children. For example, two-thirds of the children in inner city schools go without routine dental care. Many kids experience a high rate of preventable dental disease simply because their families are unable to afford sending them to a dentist for treatment. New Zealand puts dental hygienists in their public schools, and young New Zealanders have very healthy mouths regardless of their family income.

With their relatively low costs and excellent basic skills in oral health care, registered dental hygienists provide an excellent model for much greater use of independent nonphysician providers in meeting the needs of public health. Because so few doctors (dentists and physicians alike) are interested in public health, many of the public's needs for basic health care will never be met as long as qualified nonphysician providers are forced to operate under doctors' orders. In other words, freeing qualified providers from doctors' orders will likely cause more health resources to be directed to public health.

The lack of access to proper dental care is not limited to children in rural areas and the inner city, or to the elderly. Fully half of all Americans do not receive dental care on a regular basis,[9] many placing themselves at risk of various dental problems such as gum disease and tooth loss. These problems can be avoided with adequate preventive dental care and education, the core services of the dental hygienist. Of course, dentists provide the same services quite competently, but hygienists can provide them at lower cost.

Fortunately, several states already allow dental hygienists to practice independently. Their independent practices often specialize in caring for residents of nursing homes, those who are homebound, and children in schools. Dental hygienists play an important role in patient assessment and treatment, which includes routine cleanings, fluoride treatments, placing sealants, and health education. Still, many states do not grant independence to dental hygienists because dentists do not want the competition. Again, insurance reimbursement is also an impediment to independent practice. Patients have reduced access and extra cost if insurance carriers require that dental hygienists be reimbursed only through dentists.

---

9. Deborah McFall, president of the American Dental Hygienist Association. Telephone interview (April 9, 1993).

Sandra

Sandra is seven years old, and like many inner-city children her age, she is experiencing a high rate of dental cavities due to her poor diet and lack of proper oral care.

Monopoly model: The only times Sandra sees the dentist is to have her cavities filled. During these office visits she receives a regular cleaning and some instruction in dental hygiene, but this does not come on a regular basis. Since Sandra's mother receives Medicaid, there is no cost to the family for restorative dental work. However, the state is billed for each visit.

Competitive model: Sandra and her classmates see a dental hygienist who comes to their school in a mobile dental office twice a year. During these visits, qualifying students receive a thorough dental cleaning, have sealants put on their teeth to prevent decay, and are taught how to care for their teeth and mouths. The service is offered on an ability-to-pay basis, and the cost of the innovative program is shared by the state and the school system. Some students from low-income families receive the service for free. The state has determined through a number of studies that subsidized dental hygiene, early oral health screening, and dental education are much more cost-effective in the long run than restorative dental work through Medicaid and other programs.

Comparison of Average Fees		
	New Patient	Repeat Patient Without X-Rays
Dentists	$107	$50
Independent Dental Hygienists	$71	$38
Source: American Dental Hygienists' Association[10]		

---

10. "Final Report Health Manpower Pilot Project," *American Dental Hygienists' Association*, (January 1987-December 1989): 55.

Despite these difficulties, dental hygienists are pushing to expand their practice capabilities. As in professional nursing, basic education for dental hygienists is expanding from the two-year or three-year associate of arts (AA) program to a four-year, university-based program leading to a bachelor's degree.[11] In addition, all hygienists are being trained in basic emergency medical care practices such as first aid and CPR. Today's dental hygienists are intelligent and well-educated, ready to assume their traditional role in the dentist's office and to accept new roles and responsibilities elsewhere. For example, dental hygienists are moving toward certification to interpret oral x-rays. In their training and on their board exams, dental hygienists are tested on their ability to recognize abnormalities in the x-ray image. The laws of most states prohibit them from performing this function, but being able to do it will enhance their abilities to make appropriate referrals to dentists.

Many dental hygienists are trained in administering local anesthesia, but state laws restrict their ability to provide this service. The majority of the dental hygienists' work is scaling and root planing—taking plaque and calcium deposits off the teeth. This can be quite painful to some patients when done without a local anesthetic. Even though the dental hygienist performs the actual scaling and planing, all but 16 states require a dentist to apply the anesthetic. Of those remaining states, only Oregon allows dental hygienists to apply the anesthetic without the direct supervision of a dentist or physician. Thus, patients who require the procedure are forced to go to a dentist's office for their routine dental care—even where dental hygienists are allowed to practice independently. In rural areas and nursing homes, where patients rely heavily on dental hygienists, dentists are not always available to provide the required supervision. Ironically, dental hygienists in this situation must use a physician supervisor, who often has little experience in oral anesthesia, just to satisfy the state requirement. Again, assuming that the restriction is based on economics rather than the providers' certified skills, patients pay more for the service or do not get it at all.

---

11. Though the field of dental hygiene does not offer a master's or Ph.D. degree, some dental hygienists are choosing to continue their education, specializing, for example, in public health.

As compelling as these changes may seem to be, change should not come without careful, proper planning. No matter what their claims, dental hygienists wishing to practice independently should only be allowed to do so when they have proper education, licensing and certification, and are openly willing to adhere to remaining foundations of independent practice. Changing tooth structure, drilling to fill cavities, and performing oral surgery should remain in the realm of the dental doctor. Nevertheless, dental hygienists should be allowed to compete with dentists over routine, noninvasive services such as screening, cleaning, and putting sealants on teeth. Again, by enlarging the pool of qualified providers and creating competition in primarily preventive dental services, access to basic dental health care will become more available for all Americans at fair, market-driven prices.

Diagnostic Centers

The medical monopoly has not only restricted consumer access to qualified alternative providers. Based on their general premise that only a doctor is qualified to interpret the results of diagnostic tests, the medical monopoly has also denied consumers direct access to almost all medical information. Therefore, I will use the model of diagnostic centers—places where consumers can purchase certain diagnostic tests without a doctor's order—to show the potential benefits of giving consumers direct access to pertinent health information so they can become more involved in making basic decisions about their health care. Involving informed consumers—that is, consumers who have the information about their own health—is particularly appropriate now that consumers are being expected to pay a much greater share of the costs of their health care.

As we become better informed about health and illness, we should be able to purchase some basic laboratory tests (e.g., cholesterol screens and other prevention-oriented blood profiles, throat cultures, urinary analyses, etc.) directly from independent diagnostic centers. Further, the results of such basic diagnostic tests should be reported to the individual, along with reports of desirable results so that consumers will know if they should be contacting a doctor or other qualified health professional. Under the medical monopoly, only doctors are allowed to order tests, and only doctors receive the results. Consumers could save a lot of money if they could get some tests first, then decide whether they need to see a doctor. Under the current system, we have to pay the doctor first to see if we really need to see the doctor. Go figure.

While this proposal may seem futuristic, some states are already permitting consumers to order their own laboratory tests. A form of this direct-access, diagnostic-center concept was implemented in Florida in 1987, when several pharmacies in Miami started a "blood testing and results consultation service."[12] The goals of the service are to give consumers more clinical options in self-care and to contain health care costs by identifying patients at risk for cardiovascular disease. In this program, individuals have their blood pressure and weight checked and are interviewed by a phlebotomist (the trained professional who collects the sample) concerning their medical history and lifestyle. The total time for the appointment is 10 to 15 minutes. A pharmacist reviews the lab results with the patient and, if indicated, refers the patient to a physician. The pharmacists' counseling fee was $15,[13] which is a whole lot less than a doctor would charge to order the same test.

An early evaluation of the program showed that 41 percent of the participants did not have their own primary-care physician. Twenty-five percent of the participants were discovered to be at high risk for coronary heart disease, and another 40 percent were at moderate risk. The pharmacist intervened 41 percent of the time by counseling on diet, weight control, blood pressure management, stress reduction, and smoking cessation. At the same time, physicians appreciated referrals of patients requiring medical attention.[14] Not only was money saved, but care was made available to many patients who otherwise would not have received it because they did not have a doctor.

The movement for direct consumer access to medical testing is not limited to the state level. The federal government has also considered including this benefit in its programs. For example, the Health Care Financing Administration (HCFA) has noted it can save unnecessary physician fees by reimbursing

---

12. E. Clouse, "Development of a Laboratory Center in Community Pharmacies," *Florida Pharmacy Today* (May 1988): 7-8.
13. Ibid.
14. Ibid.

pre-approved, self-ordered medical tests for Medicare and Medicaid recipients, providing the practice is legal in the states where they reside.[15]

One of the great advantages of the electronic age is our ability to amass large amounts of information for individual use in education, business, entertainment, and even personal health. For example, a person receiving a test result from a diagnostic center could also receive information about the result's meaning and what actions to take. Further, modern data processing allows the interpretation of clinical information to be tied directly to the user's own medical history. In the "Charlie" scenario (page 168), the diagnostic center's computer network already has an electronic medical file on Charlie; it contains, among other things, the history of his blood sugar screenings. Charlie is notified of any deviation in his test results, and that information is automatically signaled electronically to Charlie's health care provider.

As well as being patient-specific, diagnostic centers could serve as "electronic health care libraries" where consumers could educate themselves on a wide variety of health care subjects. General patient education literature and videos would be available to help the consumer interpret test results and to act accordingly. Diagnostic centers could also sell a package of tests for consumers with special health interests or needs. For example, an independent testing facility could offer a package that gives a complete profile of the different types of cholesterol for individuals who want to improve the balance between high-density (good) and low-density (bad) lipoproteins.

Because these diagnostic centers would not be physician dependent, the price of the tests would reflect their fair market value in a competitive market. And though much of their business would be purchased out-of-pocket by consumers, insurers might well discover that covering specific consumer-purchased tests is overall less expensive than the traditional practice of reimbursing tests only through the physician.

---

15. H. Soloway, "Patient-Initiated Laboratory Testing: Applauding the Inevitable," *Journal of the American Medical Association* (October 3, 1990): 1718.

Debbie

Debbie, an accountant in her early 30s, has experienced increasing fatigue over the past few months. She's been under a lot of on-the-job stress and has had to work late most nights. As a result of her hectic schedule, she has skipped meals, often relying on the company vending machines for snacks. On Sunday, she read a newspaper article describing anemia, which reminded her that her sister was recently diagnosed with anemia due to low iron levels.

Monopoly model: Debbie makes an appointment with her family physician, describes her symptoms, and tells the doctor about her family history of low iron. The doctor performs a limited physical examination and orders an iron test, which confirms a modest degree of anemia. He gives her samples of a particular iron supplement and recommends that she buy the brand. He also reminds her to eat well-balanced meals with plenty of red meats and fresh fruits. The cost of the service is $35 for the doctor visit, $15 for the laboratory test and $4 for the iron tablets, for a total cost of $54.

Competitive model: Debbie visits a diagnostic center in a shopping center near her home and orders an iron test. She receives the results after a quick trip to the grocery store next door. The test results confirm her suspicion of a low iron level. Attached to the results is an information printout which suggests possible causes and courses of action. One of the items on the list is, of course, a recommendation to "See a health care provider." But there are other suggestions, including recommended dietary intake by food group. The printout also recommends a vitamin and mineral supplement. At a pharmacy in the same shopping center, Debbie buys a generic version of an iron-fortified vitamin and mineral supplement. The total cost of the service is $15 for the laboratory test and $8 for the multi-vitamins, for a total cost of $23.

Diagnostic centers are simply another way for consumers to receive health care without having to pay monopoly charges. In addition, giving consumers direct access to certain medical information is fully consistent with the 1990s concepts of self-responsibility and self-reliance. Diagnostic centers would be highly beneficial to the growing number of Americans who seek more control over their personal health and health care. Telemedicine—the instant access of medical information from geographically distant sources—would allow many small diagnostic centers to hook up with large medical networks, giving cheap access to the latest medical information and specialty services.

Conceivably, diagnostic centers could be located in shopping centers; within pharmacies, grocery stores, or department stores; or attached to community health or dental care clinics. In the very near future, electronic kiosks may make tests available just as automated teller machines (ATMs) make banking available on a 24-hour-a-day basis today. Only our imagination limits us in the ways we can access our own personal health care information. The potential of directly accessible diagnostic centers is just one example of how each of us can take control of our own health and become less dependent on the existing medical monopoly.

Home Health Care

Home health is another service of unquestioned value to patients and their families, but because home health services are staffed predominantly by licensed practical/vocational nurses and registered nurses who must follow doctors' orders, its potential for reducing overall expenditures on health care is diminished by its dependence on medical control. One final scenario is presented on the next page to show how the appropriate substitution of independent nonphysician providers for doctors can save money without reducing the quality of care. (In fact, I bet you will agree with me that the quality of John's care is actually better in the competitive scenario.)

By now, the reader is undoubtedly beginning to get the hang of my thinking, so I will let this scenario speak for itself as a compelling conclusion to the many arguments in favor of introducing some healthy competition into the medical marketplace.

John

When John was 21, he never thought his body would eventually give way to a progressively deteriorating disease. Going quick, he thought. That's the way he would end. But now John is 37, and he has AIDS. He knows he is in the final stages of his life, and he has chosen to live his last few months at home. Fortunately, he is in an insurance program that allows home health care and is regularly visited by a home health nurse who helps him administer his medicines and take care of personal needs. The nurse arrives one day to find John much worse than usual. He has a high fever and he seems to lapse between sleep and wakefulness.

Monopoly model: The nurse immediately calls John's physician, makes contact with the office nurse, and leaves a message for the doctor. While waiting for a return phone call, she does her best to make John comfortable. Unfortunately, she cannot stay long. Up until today, John has been doing well. And she has scheduled another patient appointment that morning. As the time draws close for her to leave, her call into the doctor still unreturned, she realizes she must do something. She informs her supervisor that she is sending John to the hospital, and over John's protests calls an ambulance. John is taken to the emergency room where he waits an hour before a physician sees him. He is immediately transferred to a critical care unit and is given a battery of tests. The doctors adjust his medication, but beyond that they realize there is nothing they can do. The nurses make him as comfortable as possible. Three days later, John dies. Five days later, John's home health nurse is called before her supervisor and is reprimanded for requesting a hospital admission without the authorization of John's doctor. The cost for John's three-day hospital stay, including the ambulance, is $7,100.

Competitive model: *The home health nurse calls her office and informs the supervisor on duty, a nurse practitioner, of John's deteriorating condition. The supervisor authorizes the home health nurse to conduct several basic tests and informs her that the field nurse practitioner is on the way. Fifteen minutes later, the nurse practitioner is at the door. Entering, she greets John with a warm smile. They know each other; she has been overseeing his care for almost two years now. John immediately brightens up, and with his usual dry wit remarks that she only visits when things get worse. "Be glad we're not married," she retorts, and John manages a laugh. Checking with the home health nurse, the nurse practitioner realizes she needs more input on John's deteriorating condition. She dials an AIDS information data bank and spells out John's situation to an AIDS specialist on the other end of the line. Receiving the information she needs, she immediately dials John's pharmacy and orders a new medication. They agree to send it over by a courier within the hour. The nurse practitioner tells the home health nurse to stay with John until further notice and phones the supervisor to find a substitute for the home health nurse's other clients for the rest of the day. The nurse practitioner and the home health nurse discuss the next steps. John will need around-the-clock, non-nursing care, at least for a while. They inform John of this and he nods. Can he get his friends and family to sit in with him? Yes, they already have agreed. John tells the home health nurse where to find the key phone numbers, and she begins to make the calls. Two weeks later, in his own home and his own bed, John dies. During the interim period, he is attended by home health nurses and non-nursing home care staff about one-third of the time. Friends and family are with him the rest. Despite the pain, John is at ease during his final days. Despite his prolonged life, the total cost for all medical and nonmedical care services in John's last two weeks are $5,400.*

Charlie

At 75, Charlie is active, involved, and very much interested in everything around him. His only real physical problem is adult onset diabetes, which he controls through proper diet and pills. A medium-built man who is very proud of his independence, he would rather spend time on his hobbies of gardening, bird-watching, and fixing bicycles for children than on, as he says, "going to the doctor like so many of these other old geezers." Nevertheless, he knows he has to be careful about his diabetic condition and realizes that his own at-home blood tests aren't always as accurate as he wishes.

Monopoly model: *Charlie makes a monthly pilgrimage to see his physician. Charlie and the doctor spend about two minutes discussing Charlie's health and about 10 minutes discussing their common outdoor interests, after which Charlie gets a blood test. While Charlie likes his doctor, he nevertheless feels a little guilty that Medicare (and the American taxpayer) picks up the tab for what he largely considers to be "a social call."*

Competitive model: *Charlie makes a monthly pilgrimage to a diagnostic center attached to his health clinic. He orders a blood test according to the health care profile that he and his geriatric nurse practitioner have generated, and review every six months or so. Charlie receives the results back within a few hours. If there are any problems, Charlie's nurse practitioner is immediately notified. Depending upon the severity of the problem, Charlie's nurse practitioner or a triage nurse from the clinic calls Charlie right away to discuss a course of action. Medicare is charged only for the blood tests and necessary clinic visits.*

Conclusion

While this focus on professions qualified for independent practice is not intended to be all-inclusive, it does provide a feasible vision of health care reform based on a patient's right to informed choice. Please note that the illustrations in this chapter are but "the tip of the iceberg." Because the number of nonphysician health professionals has grown so much—the total number of allied health professions now numbers well over 100—there is simply not enough room to mention every one and to explore its current or future qualifications for independent practice. This chapter's examples hopefully will encourage all health professions to undertake serious examination of their capabilities and to determine ways in which they can better meet consumer demand without increasing cost or reducing quality to unacceptable levels.

The case for action is clear. Revamping the entire system to allow for true choice and true competition will entail major changes at both federal and state levels of government. Let's now proceed to a four-point action plan that shows what we in this country can and must do if we are to achieve real, meaningful health reform—the kind of competitive reform that will result in greater access to less expensive health care, not just another cosmetic change in a system still controlled by doctors.

Chapter Nine

A New Prescription for Health Care Reform

The clinical history of American medical care in the last half of the twentieth century is extraordinarily impressive, but the corresponding economic history of our health care delivery system might be described as 50 years of tradition unhampered by progress.

- Clinically, the educational reforms set in motion by Abraham Flexner in 1910 effectively purged the medical profession of marginal elements. The passage of state medical practice acts eliminated most independent, nonphysician providers. Only osteopaths, podiatrists, dentists, optometrists, psychologists, and chiropractors survived the medical establishment's efforts to control all health care. Even these survivors continue to be attacked by the allopaths.

- Economically, those same reforms also laid the groundwork for the medical monopoly as it exists today. When doctors begrudgingly accepted health insurance in the 1950s because they found a way to control it—at the same time when governments, not doctors, took control of health insurance in most other countries of the Western world—the uniquely American foundation of high-cost medicine was set in place.

By forcing medical school curricula to adhere to the allopathic model, doctors trivialized all other approaches to medical care. Professions such as nursing, nurse midwifery, and physical therapy were held hostage to physicians, as was our thinking about what constitutes *health care*. What we generically call *health care* is actually *medical care*. In everyday American English, health care has come to mean what physicians do, rather than the promotion of a healthy population as a whole. True to the allopathic model, health care has come to mean aggressive intervention with drugs and surgery as both the first and last lines of defense.

Nonphysician health professionals have developed some different concepts of treatment, but their alternative approaches are suppressed as long as they are legally required to follow doctors' orders. How do we turn this troubling situation around? **Before we can make any progress, we must first embrace the concept that going to the doctor is no longer the only defensible way to meet our needs for health and medical care.**

 On the surface, medicine as it was practiced at the beginning of this century is dramatically different from the way it is practiced now. In 1900, the role of the health professional was at least as much "care" as it was "cure." In most cases, no provider could do much for the patient other than offer comfort toward one of two predictable ends: the natural process of healing or the natural process of death. A good provider, in fact, interceded as little as possible. It wasn't until the second decade of our century that Dr. Lawrence J. Henderson could write, "a random patient, with a random disease, consulting a doctor chosen at random had, for the first time in the history of mankind, a better than fifty-fifty chance of profiting from the encounter."[1]

---

1. Harold L. Blumgart, "Caring for the Patient," *New England Journal of Medicine*, 270 (1964): 449 as quoted in Rick J. Carlson's *The End of Medicine*.

The big change in medical care in the twentieth century has been our new-found ability, using the knowledge we have gained from science and the tools created by technology, to intervene in the natural processes and increase the chances of survival. "Caring" is still as important as it ever was, but it is no longer a unique function of the doctor. It can be delegated to others—allied health professionals (e.g., nurses, therapists, and psychologists), family members, the clergy, friends, teachers, and social workers. "Curing," diagnosing an illness and deciding how to treat it, has been reserved *by* the doctor as the sole domain *of* the doctor.

Although American medicine is scientifically better today than it ever was before, the doctor's curative power is still limited. In many cases, a physician's intercessions still do nothing at all and, in some cases, do harm. Medical science is far from perfect, and doctors have no basis to argue that they alone possess the knowledge to treat us properly. Doctors do not know everything there is to know about human health, and they are constantly discovering that much of what they thought they knew is wrong.

The Flexner-era reforms were quickly successful in cleaning up hospitals, providing a scientific basis for the medical school curriculum, and laying to rest much medical quackery. Today, the reasons for the Flexner reforms are no longer in existence, but the exclusionary consequences remain. Even though doctors can be justifiably proud of the cures they can effect, the net result of the turn-of-the-century reforms is that we are ending the twentieth century with an elitist, expensive, monopolistic, and inefficient medical care delivery system.

While politicians, economists, and special interest groups have presented an across-the-board spectrum of proposals for health care reform in the first year of President Clinton's term, none of these plans involves much more than developing different ways of paying for care. The basis for progress in our health care system must be more fundamental than just reforming the reimbursement system. We must realize that:

- Physicians' exclusive control over medical care is no longer justifiable because other professionals now meet the criteria of independent practice;

- Patients should be able to choose between all qualified, independent health care providers; and

- All qualified independent providers should be equally accountable under the law.

Only by realizing that we must remove health care from the exclusive control of the doctors will we be able to provide acceptable health care to more Americans at competitive prices. By following four prescriptions, our country will be able to move to a better health system for all *at lower costs with no sacrifices in quality and no new government bureaucracy.*

Prescription #1

> *State legislatures must update medical practice acts to allow qualified nonphysician providers to practice medicine independently of physicians.*

Most Americans are surprised to learn that the most fundamental power in health care—the authority to define the practice of medicine—is not at all controlled by the federal government; the licensing of health professionals is a power of the states. State legislatures have sole authority to determine what constitutes the practice of medicine and who is allowed to practice it. In the first few decades of this century, the states—many for the first time—established strict medical practice acts defining medical practice. With a few exceptions like dentists and optometrists, states gave medical doctors the authority to control health care.

In varying degrees, states have granted specific rights to other practitioners, but almost always with very strict limits on what these other practitioners could do without the direct order of a physician. More than 100 allied health professions have been recognized by various states in the past few decades, but virtually all of them are under the control of physicians for most or all of their professional activity. The reason for making everyone else subservient to the doctor has been the doctors' strenuous assertion—and who are we to challenge it, since we are not doctors—that the physician is the only person qualified to diagnose an illness and to determine the best therapy. However, *this assertion is no longer true.* The practice of medicine has become so complex that no practitioner, not even a doctor, can possess total comprehension of human health problems—witness the proliferation of specialties and sub-specialties within medicine. Many of the nonphysician providers now have more training than physicians in dealing with medical conditions within their specifically defined scope of practice.

In other words, the physician can no longer defend his position as the captain of the one and only ship. Some nonphysician providers are now qualified to become ship captains, too. They have fulfilled the same requirements that doctors previously used to establish their control over diagnosis and treatment, and states should change their state medical practice acts to allow new captains of new ships.

In order to create a marketplace where price *and* quality determine our health care purchases, states must bring their state medical practice acts up-to-date with the creation of equally qualified alternatives to medical doctors by allowing *appropriately licensed and certified* nonphysician providers to practice their specialties independent of physician control. As shown by many examples in previous chapters, these providers would be able to offer a high quality of service at a markedly lower cost if the doctor is taken "out of the loop." Just as optometrists can provide a noninvasive, lower-cost alternative to ophthalmologists, so nurse practitioners can be certified to deal with simple fractures independent of orthopedic surgeons. Likewise, respiratory therapists can recognize and treat most asthma without having to rely on a doctor's order, and in many cases a pharmacist can select the best drug—if a drug is even necessary—without needing a prescription signed by a doctor.

All these reforms could be accomplished by the creation of a model State Medical Practice Act through the National Conference of State Legislatures (NCSL). Representing all jurisdictions that define the practice of medicine, the NCSL is able to study complex issues and develop model legislation for states to adapt to their individual circumstances. In environmental protection, for example, many states have developed hazardous and solid waste programs based on model legislation prepared by the NCSL. Florida might bring in one good approach, Texas another, Oregon a third, North Carolina a fourth—all realizing that what they have is not perfect. NCSL is ideally suited to draw upon the experiences of all states, to choose the solutions that work best, and to develop a model "fill-in-the-blanks" act. Presented with a well-researched model for appropriate changes in laws that define the scope and powers of the health professions, individual state legislatures would be better prepared to enact progressive changes in important areas. The imprimatur of a prestigious national organization like NCSL would also help state legislatures resist the inevitable opposition that will be mounted by state medical societies.

The first step toward creating this model legislation is to convene an expert panel comprised of nonphysician and physician providers, hospital administrators, health economists, and other health care specialists to look at all the state practice acts affecting medicine and the other health professions. Drawing upon the existing laws of progressive states and following the foundations of independent practice as outlined in Chapter 5, the panel should be able to develop a model of an expanded, comprehensive practice act in less than a year. Once the NCSL has ratified the model act, states eager for reform and desperate to save money can use it to shape their new legislation. Again, in less progressive states where medical lobbies essentially dictate public policy, reform-minded legislators and citizen activists can hold up the model act as an example of lawmaking that has been hammered out cooperatively on a national level. The result is that real progress can be made by circumventing the special interests and partisan bickering that paralyze the U.S. Congress on health care issues.

A reexamination of the state medical practice acts is long overdue. Today's nonphysician providers are far better educated than the nonphysician providers of Flexner's day. Many nonphysician providers receive more specialized training than physicians in their particular fields. Only by rewriting these laws to reflect the realities of the 1990s and beyond can we begin to achieve our dual goal of access and affordability.

Prescription #2

*National standards must be set for licensure and certification of
all independent health care providers.*

Certainly, none of us would even think of stepping onto a commercial airliner
knowing that the pilot was neither licensed to fly nor certified to pilot our air-
craft to its destination. Even though the business end of the airline industry
was deregulated during the 1970s, the Federal Aviation Administration (FAA)
continues to maintain strict control over airline safety. The result has been an
air travel safety record in this country that is second to none in the world.
Health care can learn from this example. A brief review of some quality issues
shows why.

While physician groups will almost certainly contend that expanding the rules
governing who may practice medicine could well be an invitation to disaster,
the truth remains that under our current physician-dominated system, doctors
themselves make significant errors in the treatment of patients. I absolutely
do not make this comment as a blanket criticism of doctors because imperfec-
tion is and always will be inherent in the practice of medicine. Consequently,
physicians should not be allowed to prevent competition on the grounds that
the competitors would make some mistakes. As I said before, doctors who live
in glass houses should not throw stones.

One of the major cost problems in our health care system has been the order-
ing of useless or unnecessary treatments and medications. Indeed, the current
push to develop clinical practice guidelines derives from data showing some
doctors keep patients in the hospital longer than necessary or put patients in
hospitals when outpatient or home health care would be just as effective.
Many studies suggest that a significant proportion of all interventions ordered
by doctors may not make the patient better off, and a small number of all
physician interventions may actually be harmful to the patient. In other
words, the practice of medicine is not a perfect science, and doctors are hypo-
critical if they use arguments about quality of care to fight against direct access
to nonphysician providers who have at least as much training within carefully
defined scopes of practice.

Doctors have too long been allowed to police themselves. While the vast majority of physicians are honest and competent professionals, their inherently conflicting dual role as the exclusive provider of health care and as the exclusive judge of their own work has allowed some of them to become lax in their practice, to perform dangerous procedures for which they do not have adequate training or experience, even to continue working despite a history of major diagnostic errors or bungled operations. To its credit, the medical establishment—led by the hospital industry—has recently begun to recognize the need to certify (and recertify) physicians for the types of operations they perform and the kind of patients they treat.

There was a time in the not-too-distant past when doctors could march into a hospital and do whatever they wanted. Today, they are being asked to prove their competency periodically in given procedures before being allowed to perform them, just like commercial airline pilots must be recertified on a regular basis. (Indeed, I've often thought that doctors treating patients should be subject to random observation by peers, just as airline pilots flying commercial flights can be evaluated without warning by an FAA inspector!) The same approach can and should be used to make sure that independent nonphysician providers are also certified. Further, as states begin to apply strict guidelines for independent practice for independent nonphysician providers, doctors must be judged under the same guidelines.

Today, allopathic physicians and osteopathic physicians take the same licensing examinations in order to practice medicine. As previously noted, physicians' professional organizations, such as the American Academy of Family Practice, require an increasing amount of post-medical school continuing education for doctors to retain their certification within their medical specialty organizations. These steps are in the right direction. But in some areas of the country, physician evaluation is still left to the "old boy network," and our health care quality is suffering. Thus, opening up the independent practice of medicine to qualified nonphysician providers can and should force the states *and* the federal government to require licensing and certification of all independent health care providers, including *physicians*, based on a set of national standards.

As with the proposed process for restructuring the state medical practice acts, I believe the best approach to national standards of certification would be through the development of a national model based on systems used by states and professional societies that do a good job of insuring the competency of licensed providers. Should the states be unable to reach consensus in a reasonable time (I suggest three years), the federal government can certainly set standards—just as it has done in environmental protection, antitrust law, securities law, insurance, banking, communications, and transportation safety. After all, the FAA's success in insuring airline safety is exemplary, and contrary to what some might think, dying at the hands of an incompetent surgeon operating beyond his abilities is far more probable than dying in a commercial aviation accident.

One of the unwritten rules of a monopoly is that its members protect not only the monopoly itself, but fellow members of the monopoly. Physicians are no exception. While our current system has generally worked well and most physicians are admirably conscientious in doing the best job possible, many doctors have been guilty of providing poor care, and too many of their mistakes have been swept under the rug. *Quality control*, not physician autonomy, must be the key element in determining the universal standards of independent health care practice. I am certainly not saying that independent nonphysician providers will necessarily be any better than physicians. I am saying that I have no reason to believe they will be any worse, and that all independent providers need to be regulated according to the same state-mandated procedures.

This prescription does not necessarily mean that the states must do the certifying. The professionals' own organizations could be held legally and financially responsible for the conduct of their members under state or federal guidelines and according to general norms set across all independent health care disciplines. The result would be greater objectivity and more meaningful recertification of providers with the least amount of government intrusion.

Prescription #3

Health insurance reform should mandate reimbursement to all qualified health professionals, with payment to any qualified professional limited to the reasonable charge of the least-cost qualified provider (LCQP).

When physicians first set up Blue Cross and Blue Shield programs, their purpose was as much protective as it was altruistic. Seeing the rise of the private health insurance industry, they took the advice of the old adage, "If you can't beat 'em, join 'em," and launched their own plan. The key to their defensive involvement was *control*—specifically, the fear of losing it. Taking the position that no third party should come between the physician and his patient, doctors championed the idea that the physician must be free of financial constraints in order to practice the art and science of the profession in the patients' best interest.

I have already discussed how and why doctors initially fought the rise of private health insurance, only to embrace it when they discovered they could own the dominant carrier. The newfound ability to control health insurance meant not only control over who was going to deliver health care, but control over its prices as well. Doctors benefited early on by writing into the Blue Cross and Blue Shield programs *their right to set fees* without any outside intervention, be it from the free market or otherwise.

Because of the strength of the doctor-controlled plans, this "right" effectively carried over to the private insurance companies. The other third parties quickly learned that if doctors were not paid what they wanted, doctors could simply refuse to take care of patients covered by the private plans. In 1965, when the federal government created Medicare and Medicaid, doctors further solidified their power to determine their own fees by convincing the federal government to select the doctor-controlled Blue Cross and Blue Shield plans to be the programs' financial intermediary.

While the federal government is leading a shift from reimbursing physicians based on "usual, customary, and reasonable" (UCR) charges to the Resource-Based Relative Value System (RBRVS), this change still does not represent a competitive market reform. *The only way medical care is going to become affordable is to peg government reimbursement to the charge of the least-cost qualified provider for any given service.* Further, to insure an efficient and competitive outcome, the group of qualified providers must be expanded to include independent nonphysician providers as well as physicians.

Health insurance plans should not have to pay a physician's fee when an equally qualified nonphysician is able to provide the same service at a lower, competitive price. Health insurance should limit reimbursement to an amount equal to a reasonable fee of the least expensive health professional who is qualified to provide a specific medical service, in much the same way that traditional UCR-based plans have limited payment to the 90th percentile of all fees submitted by doctors. Reasonableness could be determined by a methodology similar to the one used to set RBRVS payments.

At the same time, the system must *not* prevent patients from paying the difference when they want to get care from a more expensive source (a practice known as balance billing). For example, if the fee for a routine office visit is $40 for a physician and $25 for a nurse practitioner, insurance would pay $25 to either provider. The patient who prefers to see the physician will have to pay the $15 difference out-of-pocket, subject to the policy's coinsurance and deductible provisions. (The physician might eventually get the point of competition and find a way to lower his fee!) Likewise, if a physician charges $45 for a service that costs $55 when provided by a physical therapist, the physical therapist's insurance reimbursement would be limited to $45. The point is to build some consumer cost-consciousness into the third-party reimbursement system—not to penalize doctors.

The ramifications of this shift from fees set by doctors—known in economic theory as price leadership—to fees set by competition will be far-reaching. Once programs for training independent nonphysician providers have been expanded and the qualified nonphysicians have begun to occupy their proper place in the health care marketplace, third parties can expect to cut their costs by significant amounts without cutting benefits—all by buying in a competitive market from least-cost suppliers. Significant savings will also be realized by consumers. The expected size of the savings cannot be known with any precision since we do not have any widespread experience with the competitive approach—just as the Congressional Budget Office cannot begin to know the potential savings, if any, of the Clinton Plan because its bureaucratic structure has never existed. Nevertheless, existing income differentials lead me to a first-order approximation of potential savings in the range of 10 percent to 30 percent.

Governments need look no further than the prescription drug market for a promising example of their power to cut health care costs by refusing to pay for name-brand drugs when a generic drug is just as good. The pharmaceutical sector of the health care industry has become quite competitive since government took the lead in refusing to pay the prices of prescription drugs when generics were available.

The economic wisdom of only providing insurance coverage, when appropriate, for the least-expensive providers has already been learned by some of the country's most financially sound health maintenance organizations. For example, in the highly successful Kaiser-Permanente system, one in every three patient contacts is with a nonphysician provider. Even higher rates of substituting less expensive but equally qualified nonphysician providers are found in the U.S. military. Successful health maintenance organizations and the health services of our armed forces prove that money can be saved by refusing to pay for a doctor when a non-doctor will do just fine.

Government should take the lead in achieving the same savings in all sectors of the health economy by immediately restricting insurance reimbursement to a reasonable fee charged by the least-cost qualified provider. As shown in the discussions of virtually every nonphysician provider (Chapters 6 and 7), requiring mandatory reimbursement to all qualified providers will also be essential so that physicians cannot subvert the competition by preventing insurance from paying for otherwise lawful care.

When we de-monopolize health care by opening it up to qualified practitioners other than physicians, we must also free it from the inherent price-fixing formalized by doctors when they effectively took control of the health insurance industry. While the Resource-Based Relative Value System has attempted to address some of the inequities within that system, RBRVS does absolutely nothing to end physicians' unjustifiable control over all medical practice. Only by allowing prices to float in a free market of all qualified providers—and restricting third-party payments to the lowest of those levels—will we begin to approach affordable health care for all.

Prescription #4

Government funding for medical research and education must be reallocated from expensive and marginally unproductive physician-dominated programs to programs that increase the supply of independent, nonphysician providers.

In the late 1960s, Rashi Fein's influential book, *The Doctor Shortage*, not only launched a national "crash" program to educate more doctors, it also encouraged states and the federal government to spend more money on educating "mid-level providers"—the medical establishment's subtly derogatory term for nurse practitioners, physicians' assistants (PAs), and other allied health providers. The reigning belief at the time was that the country was facing a cataclysmic doctor shortage—a crisis of major proportions—and that while the country waited anxiously for the nation's medical schools to turn out a new and significantly larger supply of American doctors, mid-level providers would have to be trained as an interim solution to meeting the country's immediate health care needs.

For a number of years, the U.S. had been importing foreign doctors to fill the perceived gap. In addition, American students who could not get into our country's medical schools were training in foreign medical schools and returning home to set up relatively lucrative practices in the United States. But these solutions were often unsatisfactory. Many Americans balked at being treated by physicians whose ethnicity, culture, and accent were different from their own. Furthermore, foreign-educated doctors, be they foreign nationals or native-born Americans, were not as uniformly well-trained as their American-educated counterparts. There was also a compelling moral argument that the countries training and exporting their native doctors were in much greater need of their services than was the United States.

Thus, policy makers responding to the expected physician shortage determined that American-trained, mid-level providers (or physician extenders, as they were also called at the time) were a better long-run solution to the inadequate supply of doctors. They could be educated more quickly than doctors, be trained to do many of the doctors' more menial tasks, and, presumably, take orders just like nurses. Furthermore, educating mid-levels was relatively inexpensive—about one-sixth of the cost of educating a physician.

In a short period of time these programs became quite successful, with prestigious medical schools leading the way in the development of allied health programs. Physicians and policy makers additionally saw the "mid-level" as a solution to one of the most fundamental problems in our health care system: the maldistribution of physicians. Thus, this new breed of health care professional was dispatched to our country's inner cities and rural areas to handle the tasks the physicians didn't want to do themselves—to serve the urban poor and people in areas where physicians didn't want to live. For example, several states allow nurse practitioners to operate rural or inner-city clinics without having a doctor present on the presumption that some health care is better than no health care at all. (As I mentioned earlier, I am offended by this thinking. If mid-level means mid-quality, my rural neighbors and I don't want it.)

Nonphysician providers have proven their comparable worth and their ability to stand on their own. Since they have also proven to be economical, we need to increase their supply just as aggressively as we sought to eliminate the doctor shortage 25 years ago. *If we cannot come up with new funds to create the needed supply of nonphysician providers, then taking money away from medical schools will be a necessary and worthwhile trade-off because nonphysician providers are needed now more than doctors.* In other words, we now face the prospects of a nonphysician provider shortage every bit as serious as the doctor shortage predicted in the late 1960s, and we must be just as committed to solving it.

While these new "mid-level" programs worked in theory and in practice for at least a short time (mostly the 1970s), physicians soon concluded that creating this new breed of health care professional was somewhat like creating a Frankenstein's monster—it wanted a life of its own. Physicians were thus forced to respond accordingly. A common response was to declare victory in the "War on the Doctor Shortage," thus alleviating the need to commit major funds to the programs for training nonphysician providers. Doctors' support for allied health training quickly began to disappear.

However, organized medicine never really had to play its hand because the Reagan era began just about the time all the new medical schools were up and running. The budget ax fell most heavily on the fledgling training programs for nonphysician providers because these cuts would affect doctors the least. Before it was all over, damages extended beyond mid-level and allied health education programs. Health care programs that relied most heavily on non-physician providers, such as community health centers and the National Health Service Corps, also failed to get expected levels of funding for several years.

The Bottom Line

In order to accomplish the goal of de-monopolizing the doctor-driven medical care system, a concerted effort must be made to reallocate funds from expensive research and education programs for physicians to less costly programs designed for nonphysician providers (assuming that new funds will not be made available in today's budget-conscious environment). The 1980s cuts in funding to schools that trained nonphysician providers did much to curtail the supply of these allied health care professionals just as they were developing skills for independent practice. In the early 1980s, for example, there was an oversupply of registered physical therapists (RPT). Today, the few schools that are still educating RPTs cannot produce enough graduates to fill the demand, and physical therapists' salaries are rising dramatically. The reason is because many physical therapy education programs are associated in one way or another with medical schools. When the Reagan-era budget cuts hit the medical schools, the physicians in charge naturally found it easier to do away with physical therapy programs than with the programs that trained doctors.

At the same time, progressive health systems that have discovered the true value of nonphysician providers (e.g., Kaiser-Permanente and our armed forces) have been hiring large numbers of them. The result is that nonphysician providers are in incredibly short supply. We must dramatically increase their numbers before relative scarcity causes their incomes to approach those of physicians. Investing in more nonphysician providers capable of competitive independent practice—*even if it means investing in fewer physicians*—is one of the most intelligent moves we could make toward achieving the desired improvements in our nation's health care: lower costs, more access, and acceptable quality.

Reforming the educational priorities of the medical education system must follow a multipronged approach. First, a major effort should be made to attract top-quality faculty to the educational programs that train independent nonphysician providers. Because of the emphasis on educating the physician at the expense of other health care providers, there simply has not been enough funding to expand the academic and research base in the allied health care fields. Thus, there is currently a shortage of doctoral-trained faculty available to teach in the allied health schools. Good teachers are available, but they must be wooed away from medical schools and universities until more doctorates can be generated within the nonphysician disciplines themselves.

At the same time, funds must be made available for research within the academic disciplines of the nonphysician providers. The majority of medical research today is being done by physicians and clinical scientists on medical school faculties. This fact inherently skews the research focus toward the doctor's model of disease and treatment. For example, as our population grows older, the attention should shift from how to fix the damaged or aging body to how to live a happy, healthy life within that body. This is an area where research in the nonphysician models, with their more holistic clinical paradigms, is a much-needed investment in our future.

This progress cannot be accomplished until programs for educating the nonphysician professionals are put on equal footing with medical school programs, removing physicians' control over the nonphysician programs. This approach does not necessarily mean removing allied health programs from medical schools; I know from firsthand experience the two can work side by side as long as they are not fighting each other for funding. Therefore, it does mean earmarking state and federal funds separately according to needs and demand, without the possibility of physicians controlling the programs for training nonphysician providers.

When Congress and the states chose in the late 1960s to double our national investment in medical schools in order to deal with the feared doctor shortage, programs for nonphysician providers grew to a large extent because of the "trickle down" effect—a phenomenon that ended with the Reagan administration. To meet the current crisis in health care, Congress and the states must renew and expand a commitment to the competing programs, providing them with their own deserved legitimacy and independence. We must take away the doctor's authority to order the health system according to his will. We will all benefit when our educational programs make sure he gets some needed competition.

Chapter Ten

How Will We Know When We Get There If We Don't Know Where We're Going?

Those who do not understand the lessons of history are doomed to repeat it.

Santana

Nothing is as powerful as an idea whose time has come.

Victor Hugo

When the state medical practice acts gave control of the health care franchise to university-trained doctors, the entire scope of medicine could be encompassed by one person. Medical science had a relatively undeveloped understanding of the human body, and doctors did not have much technology to master. Stethoscope, thermometer, and microscope were about the extent of a physician's diagnostic tools, so the little black bag could hold all the equipment and become the symbol of American medicine.

As Abraham Flexner so graphically pointed out, doctors who were educated in the few scientifically-oriented medical schools were at the time the only medical practitioners who had the appropriate training to offer treatment with some consistent, verifiable success. However, in the ensuing 75 years, medicine has become so incredibly complex that even top-flight medical school professors must struggle to keep abreast of all the latest developments. Today, no one person could possibly know everything there is to know about medicine, and the traditional black bag isn't even big enough to hold the laptop computer that is fast becoming an essential tool for the modern doctor.

As I often say in my speeches about the future of health care, medical science and technology are changing so fast that it takes a good doctor an incredible amount of time and effort just to stay confused. Judging from the response of my audiences—often including physicians who nod supportively when I make this statement—the doctor can no longer know it all. Specialization not only makes sense; it is absolutely essential. That we should lament the passing of the all-knowing generalist in medicine—the archetypal family doctor of the 1950s—is frankly naïve because physicians have had to become specialists. In consequence, doctors in the last half of the twentieth century have become quite used to sharing the overall responsibility for treating patients or populations—but so far, only with other doctors. Now is the time for us as a nation to recognize that some of the new, fully qualified specialists will not be doctors.

Very few, if any, doctors would dispute the statement that the majority—probably a good deal more than half—of all initial patient contacts do not require the skills of a provider with 12 to 15 years of specialized post–high-school education (the training of today's medical doctor). For example, I see the nurse practitioner, working either independently or in collaborative practice with other physician and nonphysician providers, becoming the twenty-first century equivalent of the American family doctor of the mid-1900s. Trained with a patient-centered focus and steeped in the nursing model of caring and nurturing, the advanced practice nurses are at least as qualified as the research-focused, disease-oriented allopathic doctors to deal with ordinary aches, pains, colds, flus, and checkups. They are arguably even more qualified to address the nation's needs for health promotion and disease prevention—the long-run keys to reducing medical care spending as a percent of the gross national product! Like many of the other nonphysicians qualified for independent practice, they are ready to meet our need for primary care.

First Things First: Primary Care

As this chapter's title implies, our quest for health reform is not proceeding with a clear and shared goal in mind. We have devoted so much effort to our obsession with problems of the current system that we haven't taken time to develop a national consensus of what a better system would look like. Opportunistic politicians have orchestrated a steady stream of sad stories about people who did not have insurance to pay for expensive treatments, but the main solution proposed by our leaders—universal coverage—hardly seems like true reform to me. Giving everyone insurance "that would always be there" (President Clinton's promotional phrase) would only increase peoples' ability to pay for the inefficient system we already have, thereby increasing the total costs of health care even more.

I prefer to approach reform by imagining a cost-effective system we could create rather than cataloging the economic inefficiencies of the system we have. We need to approach the problem like engineers, not accountants. Engineers are trained to define the problem, to imagine a viable solution, and then to work back from the solution to the problem to figure out how we can get from where we are (the problem) to where we want to be (the solution).[1] Engineers are paid to be creative, to imagine things being different. Assign the same problem to 100 engineers and you may get more than 100 different solutions! Accountants, on the other hand, are trained to use standardized financial procedures to describe the flow of dollars through a business. Accountants are not paid to be creative. Give the same accounting problem to 100 accountants, and they are all supposed to come up with the same answer. We need both engineers and accountants to run our businesses, but engineering provides the better conceptual model for health reform.

Sadly, our political leaders seem to think almost exclusively like accountants; I have not heard them say much about how our problems could be solved by reengineering the delivery system. The congressional approach to health reform is analogous to refinancing a company's debt to solve deep-seated problems with management or production—something like using junk bonds to provide more cash for "business as usual" rather than replacing poor managers

---

1. People who make public policy ought to be required to read a good book about the theory and practice of engineering. I recommend *Conceptual Blockbusting* by James Adams (New York: Addison-Wesley, 1990).

or modernizing an old plant. Finance and accounting are important, but they cannot overcome deeper systemic problems. For example, we could impose capitation—a central concept in most reform plans—and still see our health expenditures continue to rise (see sidebar: "Capitation vs. Managed Care").

I believe that the major structural flaw of our health care system—the problem that must be solved in order to reinvent it—is the oversupply of medical specialists. *If we really want to end up with a less-expensive health care system that is accessible to more people, we must purposefully engineer a reallocation of resources from specialty care to primary care.* In the United States, approximately two-thirds of our physicians are medical specialists who treat organ-specific or system-specific diseases; only one-third are primary care practitioners who treat the whole patient. The ratio is just the opposite in the countries whose lower costs and better health we envy.

If we are really serious about getting more for the money we spend on health services, we had also better get real serious real soon about providing more primary care. This means providing less specialty care unless we want to devote even more of our gross national product to health care, which I seriously doubt. As candidate, Bill Clinton promised he would cut medical expenditures as a portion of GNP. As President, he has promoted a health care plan that would increase health care spending from approximately 14 percent to 18 percent of our economy. Much of the dramatic decline in public support for his plan can be attributed to President Clinton's failure to deliver what candidate Clinton promised. Americans do not want to spend more on health care. They want better value for the money they do spend.

For several reasons, increasing the supply of accessible and affordable primary care is the key to reaching the goal of better value.

- First, primary care practitioners deal with our medical problems when they are still minor—at the early stages when illness and injury can be treated most cost-effectively and when complications can be prevented. Many patients who have expensive medical problems requiring a specialist's care are people who did not seek help from a primary care provider at the onset of symptoms. If we want to reduce how much we spend on expensive specialty care, we must create a health system that makes primary care readily available when people need it.

- Second, primary care practitioners treat the whole person. They are trained to think comprehensively about the patient, not just the patient's clinical condition. They address health promotion and disease prevention in addition to dealing with medical problems in the early stages. Good primary care practitioners establish an ongoing relationship with each patient so they can identify and address long-term problems in an individual's health. (In contrast, medical specialists are trained to think about very narrow clinical problems—which is a good thing. We do need specialists, just not so many of them.)

- Third, primary care practitioners are the ideal "gatekeepers" for the entire health care delivery system (for example, deciding when a patient does or does not need to be seen by a specialist). They can coordinate referrals to multiple specialists when necessary and interpret specialists' findings in accord with the patient's overall health history and concepts of health. Having a gatekeeper makes a lot of sense and potentially saves a lot of money. Each of us ought to insist on having one, and it should definitely be a primary care professional who is skilled at seeing the "big picture."

- Last, but not least, people want primary care. I've been personally involved in health surveys of more than 25,000 individuals over the past 10 years, and I've found that consumers want affordable and accessible primary care more than anything else. Indeed, for every sad story about someone whose insurance would not cover treatment for a rare disease, I've heard hundreds of equally frustrated people tell how they could not get treated for an everyday health problem because primary care was not available to them. Many of them end up going to the emergency room when the problem gets worse—ultimately costing the system several times as much as a primary care visit.

Fortunately, as shown by the scenarios in earlier chapters of this book, we now have several types of nonphysician providers who are well qualified to deliver primary care. These professionals who can help solve our problem are already waiting in the wings, ready for us to bring them to the center of the economic stage to compete directly with the doctors who no longer deserve to have the spotlight all to themselves. Let's finish our analysis by seeing how the history of medical care in the United States is consistent with a creative vision of a different health care system.

Capitation vs. Managed Care

Capitation and managed care are among the most often-heard buzzwords of the debate over health reform. They are frequently—and wrongly—used as synonyms. Some capitation plans do not manage care, and some plans that do manage care are not capitated. Treating these two different concepts as the same thing is a sign of the confusion that occurs when we focus on paying for health care rather than producing it more efficiently.

Capitation is a method of paying for care. In contrast to the fee-for-service method staunchly defended by organized medicine, capitation is a contractual payment system that gives providers a fixed amount per person (per capita) to deliver a defined package of benefits to a specific population. The advantages of capitation include fixing total costs of care in advance and simplifying the payment process (for example, eliminating the complex and expensive system needed to process millions of fee-for-service claims).

Managed care is a method of monitoring the care that is delivered, using outcomes-based practice guidelines to ensure that the right things are done at the right time, and, conversely, to guard against the use of medical resources that do not contribute to the desired outcome. Some doctors express their dislike for managed care by calling it "cookbook medicine," so I prefer to think of it instead as the medical equivalent to an airplane pilot's checklist.

Paradoxically, capitation and managed care can work at cross purposes. The fixed budget imposed by capitation can create incentives to minimize the amount of care delivered. On the other hand, a good managed-care system based on clinical standards could promote the delivery of services that might not be provided under a capitated system based on financial imperatives. Assuming that we cannot afford all the care we want, we must prepare to make intelligent trade-offs between our desire to save money and our desire to get good care. If we ever have to choose between capitation and managed care, I'll take managed care.

Lessons of History

I have always been impressed by the wisdom of Santana's famous dictum about the value of understanding history so that we are not doomed to repeat it. Unfortunately, many people misinterpret the quote, ending up instead with a statement to the effect that history runs in cycles. Well, what goes around probably will come around again if we fail to see what we can learn from the past, so I have spent considerable time trying to identify relevant lessons of history during my 25 years of teaching, researching, and consulting in the health care industry. (Here's where being a health care futurist comes in handy.)

In the interests of leaving the reader with some optimistic conclusions and interesting challenges about a future of health care that is better than the past we are trying so desperately to reform, here are four lessons of history that should inspire us to think big if we really want to change our health care delivery system for the better—that is, do something more exciting than just find new ways to pay the doctor.

Lesson #1: The health care delivery system in the United States is remarkably flexible. As you look back on the previous chapters in this book, think about how much things have changed in the American health care system since the foundations of modern medical care were laid in the mid-1800s. Medical science has undergone several revolutionary redefinitions. Infectious diseases were understood and conquered in the late 1800s and the early 1900s. With most people then able to survive into old age, doctors turned their attention to treating degenerative conditions like heart disease and cancer with considerable success—just look at the dramatic increases in life expectancy over the last half of the twentieth century. The hospital has been redefined, from a place for poor people to die to a place for anyone to be restored to health. Sadly, for those who do die, the causes of death have changed. Fifty years ago, we feared death from polio, heart attacks, and cancer. Today's leading killers include tobacco, AIDS, and violence. Health insurance came out of nowhere in the early part of this century to become the main source of payment for health care. Yes, health care changes a lot in the United States; it is a vibrant sector of our economy.

Lesson #2: Change can come fast and unexpectedly. Many of the changes that led to Lesson #1 came almost out of nowhere. Many of the most significant advancements in medical science came from unexpected discoveries like penicillin and modern genetics. Organized medicine's strenuous opposition to health insurance disappeared in very short order once doctors learned how to tame the beast. President Johnson was able to secure the passage of Medicare and Medicaid laws in 1965 after President Kennedy had been unsuccessful in attempts to do the same just two years earlier. Congress created the Prospective Payment System in 1983; the legislation was not even discussed in 1982. Last, but not least, the Catastrophic Health Insurance Act didn't last two months in the early 1990s when senior citizens learned that they were being expected to pay for the program. No, our system is not always stuck on tradition; it is not "cast in stone." It can respond rapidly to new possibilities—when it wants to!

Lesson #3: No one is in long-run control of our health care system. I think we are inclined to believe that someone, most likely the American Medical Association (AMA), is the power behind the scenes in directing the evolution of our health care delivery system. Well, the events chronicled in this book suggest that the AMA has a pretty good history of learning how to make the best of undesired outcomes, but look at how much of the evolution of our health care system was originally opposed by organized medicine. Governments, both state and federal, have become major players in the health care game over the past 30 years, but they are totally frustrated in their lack of ability to get what they want from the system. The consumer isn't really king, either. Of course, doctors have preserved their monopoly over diagnosis and treatment for the past 60 to 70 years, but I do not know a single doctor who feels in control right now. Indeed, I cannot think of a single interest group that gets everything it wants, which is a sign that no one group is in control of the system.

When I talk to hospital and medical groups, I add a fourth lesson, namely that flexibility is the key to success as a provider. However, since this book is written more for consumers than for providers, I prefer to conclude my review of history with a challenge rather than a lesson. If we have a flexible system capable of changing fast because no one has enough long-run control to prevent the rise of an idea whose time has come, then consumers should feel empowered to express their vision of a different future.

The good news is *consumers can bring about desired change if they will just get together and let lawmakers know that they want a competitive health care system, one where they are free to choose among qualified alternative providers.* I know that consumers are not used to speaking up when it comes to health care, but there has never been a better time to do so.

Visions of the Future

As soon as I began to understand the lessons of history in health care, I felt liberated in the quest to rethink—indeed, to reinvent—health care. (As implied in the Preface, I probably began to challenge the established order when I read Dr. Seuss as a child and *Mad* magazine as a teenager. It's only an accident of history that I ended up being a contrarian in the health industry.) I also know from many years of teaching health planning that we are very likely to follow an aimless path if we do not know where we want to go.

In the interests of establishing some direction for a consumer revolution in health care, I present my vision of a different and better health care delivery system. I absolutely do not contend that this reinvented view is the one and only path to improvement. The reader should not feel that the only choice is between my view and the established order. The future offers far more possibilities than I can imagine, so I will be most pleased if my vision causes others to do their own rethinking and produce even better concepts for improving health care in the United States. Then we can have a relaxed and thoughtful dialog about real health care reform—not the narrow, disappointing, and rushed discussion that has occupied Washington thus far in 1994.

- *Independent nonphysician providers will deliver a significant portion of our nation's primary care.* Because our nation has neither the time nor the money to expect medical schools to meet our enormous needs for basic health services, nurse practitioners will be the key resource for filling the primary care gap left by physicians moving more and more into specialized care. Nurse practitioners trained in family, pediatric, geriatric, and long-term care will complement family practitioners as the backbone of our nation's health care system—both as competitors in nurse-only practices and as partners with doctors in collaborative practices (a nice new choice for consumers to have). Nurse midwives will take over many of the primary care functions of obstetrician/gynecologists, including complete management of low-risk pregnancies. Pharmacists will assume a more active role in assisting customers with self-diagnosis and self-treatment. Optometrists will provide the great majority of primary eye care. Physical therapists will be much more involved in dealing directly with patients and will be the initial contact for muscle-related injury and rehabilitation. Audiologists and respiratory therapists will similarly take a larger role in treating individuals with hearing and breathing difficulties, respectively. In oral health care, dental hygienists will offer teeth cleaning and examination services independent from dentists. Doctors (both physicians and dentists) will continue to do everything they have been doing, but they will no longer have "the only game in town." Consumers will be able to get care much more conveniently and affordably.

• *Pharmacies and diagnostic centers will offer consumers new opportunities for self-diagnosis and self-treatment.* Just as the full-service gas station has given way to the self-service "quick stop," so will pharmacies and diagnostic centers provide a less expensive and more convenient alternative for consumers who feel sufficiently well-informed to deal initially and preventively with their own health care needs. Computer information terminals in pharmacies will help consumers find answers to questions regarding both health and illness. Pharmacists themselves will be skilled at diagnosing common ailments like throat infections and skin rashes with the help of computer protocols and over-the-counter diagnostic tools. Through computer networks, consumers will be able to authorize pharmacists to access their personal medical records in order to check for allergies to prescription drugs or other medications. Consumers will be able to walk into diagnostic centers located in pharmacies, health care clinics, shopping malls, supermarkets, and department stores for blood tests, urinalyses, throat cultures, and even some x-rays. Diagnostic centers will be electronically linked to large, fully equipped laboratories for backup support and confirmation of diagnoses and to health care databases storing consumer medical records. Diagnostic centers and pharmacies will both offer educational services to consumers by providing interactive computer programs and video libraries.

• ***The market for primary care services will develop to resemble the market for other consumer goods and services.*** The new providers and new services will increasingly operate in retail locations. (I've coined the phrase, "healer dealer," to describe the entrepreneur who will bring about this revolution in the medical marketplace.) Medical "stores" will vary in size from small, basic-care operations located in shopping malls and freestanding buildings to large "megaclinics" offering everything from dentistry and family medical care to physical therapy and lifesaving emergency services. In comparison with today's typical provider, the new medical retailers will be much more attuned to the needs of consumers. Most clinics of the future will be open during the daytime and evening and on weekends because so many consumers will prefer expanded hours to the traditional "9 to 5" hours of doctors' offices. Education and prevention will be major product lines of the retail health and medical stores of the future. The larger locations will also offer comprehensive wellness programs promoting healthy lifestyles and will provide facilities for teaching nutrition and proper exercise. Many will be linked to health clubs with gymnasiums, workout rooms, and even swimming pools. The thrust of the new clinics will be as much keeping people healthy as diagnosing and treating people who are ill. The dream of comprehensive care will become a reality for customers who choose to buy from these new health stores.

• ***Physicians will assume the roles of both specialty-care providers and entrepreneurs within the new system.*** Doctors have survived every change within health care, and I see no reason why the revolution of my vision should put them out of business. In fact, after some loud grumbling about the inconvenience of one more attack on their authority, I fully expect that many physicians will be quiet leaders in setting up the new system. (I have *enormous* respect for the many physicians I know who are developing new approaches to the delivery of medical care, and I am proud of my associations with the two national programs that are leading the way in training the physician executives and entrepreneurs of the future.) Believe me, doctors really are smart and talented people. Monopoly is an economic behavior, not a personality defect. Doctors will not all sit idly by as they begin to comprehend the business opportunities represented by the rise of independent nonphysician providers. Although they will be sharing their clinical role as the nation's primary care provider, doctors will continue to provide specialized care for acute and chronic illness.

• *Basic public health services will be delivered in many new settings.* Schools will provide part-time pediatric and dental care services employing nurse practitioners and dental hygienists, particularly in traditionally underserved areas like rural America and inner cities. "Healthmobiles" staffed by nurse practitioners, nurse midwives, and dental hygienists will also bring primary medical care and dental services to special locations like farm worker camps, nursing homes, and retirement communities. To compete with the new full-service medical clinics, dental offices will also begin to offer basic health care screening for problems like hypertension and eating disorders. As the population grows older, Americans will receive more long-term health care in their homes. Electronic monitoring machines will be attached to telephones to allow those who are homebound to relay medical information to clinics or home health care services. Patient education will be a major component in getting the homebound to take care of their own health care needs. Nurse practitioners will largely replace doctors as the primary care providers in nursing homes and home health programs, while doctors will move more towards consultative relationships with the nurse practitioners. More and more follow-up will be done by telephone as reimbursement systems switch from fee-for-service to managed care and capitation.

• *Voluntary (tax-exempt) hospitals will assume new and different roles as the institutional center of the future health care system.* The hospital as a physical facility (that is, as a big brick building with beds in it) will still be the place to go for emergency medical services and treatment of the most complex and specialized medical procedures. However, the hospital as a business entity will evolve to become the general contractor of the health care system. If for no other reason than its superior access to the large amounts of money that will be needed to develop fully integrated delivery systems, the hospital is better positioned than any other provider to be at the center of the health industry in the not-too-distant future—by the end of the century, I think.

Another reason for the likely leadership of the hospital is its superior capability to bear institutional liability and to manage risk. Once hospitals learn how to manage outpatient care and how to integrate clinical and financial information into one database—goals they are now diligently pursuing—they will also know more about medical care delivery than any other business entity in the health industry. Money and knowledge add up to power, so hospitals have a bright future to my way of thinking. Not too many years from now, the majority of independent providers (including doctors, nurse practitioners and midwives, pharmacists, therapists, etc.) will be employees of hospitals, and doctors who have abandoned clinical practice will be among the most successful chief executives in the industry. When all this happens, we will need to make sure that the hospital industry does not itself become monopolistic. However, I believe that voluntary hospitals—community, religious, and other tax-exempt organizations—are preparing themselves nicely for a leadership role that is theirs to lose. The Internal Revenue Service has recently made the continuation of tax-exempt status contingent on a hospital's ability to prove that the community it serves is better off because of the hospital. I am not worried about the future of health care as long as hospitals see their mission not as earning a profit, but as meeting the community's needs as efficiently as possible.

And Now, for Something Completely Different . . .

During the latter part of the nineteenth century and into the twentieth, the thrust of government policy was to put the doctor squarely in the driver's seat of our health care delivery system. From the 1930s until the present day, the assumption underlying virtually all health-reform proposals has been that doctors were the heart of that system. Doctors may have lost considerable control over the payment mechanism, but they have maintained control over the care of patients because we have not recently reexamined their ultimate authority over other members of the health care delivery team.

No matter what options we consider for national health care reform—whether they be changes in insurance law, managed competition, or a single-payer system—none will fully come to grips with our system's fundamental economic problem: the absence of true competition among providers. Even if one of the current reform proposals should pass, we would still be saddled with the economic problems of clinical monopoly.

I have used "the captain of the ship" metaphor to explain this monopoly. Since the metaphor itself derives from transportation, the transportation industry provides a fitting illustration of the economic lesson that should now be applied to health care. At the time of the Flexner Report, railroads had an effective monopoly over transportation throughout the United States; they also had an incredible amount of political power.

If the railroad barons had thought like the physicians of the time, they could have sought to outlaw passenger cars and airplanes on the grounds that these alternative forms of transportation were unsafe and unscientific—an arguably defensible position in 1910. Fortunately, the railroads did not have this inclination. But if they had, they probably would have maintained tight control over development of the automobile and airline industries, and we would now be arguing the need to break up the railroads' control over airlines and automobile manufacturers so that consumers could have truly competitive choices among alternative forms of proven transportation.

We obviously need to reinvent our country's health care delivery system. This means rethinking all its underlying assumptions and imagining different ways of getting things done. We must rebuild it using all the resources that are available to us at the end of the twentieth century, not just those that were available to us at the beginning. We should also draw upon one of the under-lying strengths of our nation—economic competition—now that alternatives are available to us.

But before we proceed with setting the course for the next several decades, we must also ask ourselves one very important question: *What do we ultimately want from our health care system?*

    (a) Less expensive health care.

    (b) Higher-quality health care.

    (c) Health care for all Americans.

    (d) All of the above.

To this day, we delude ourselves by thinking that the obvious answer is (d). "All of the above" is not an acceptable answer in an era of limited resources. We need to make a choice because we simply cannot have it all. Top-quality, least-cost health care for everyone is an impossibility. Politicians may talk like we can have it all, but good economists know better. You do not have to be a rock-et scientist to realize that improving the quality of care adds to its cost or that extending health care to all residents also means spending more, not less. On the other hand, to spend less on health care in a system without competition, we will need to reduce quality or provide fewer services—real-world trade-offs that our politicians have not been willing to discuss in the public debate over health care reform. (I could use calculus and the economic model of con-strained optimization to prove this point, but I will spare you the detail. Consult any good intermediate textbook in microeconomic theory if you need mathematical proof.)

Ironically, the answer that I think we would all accept is one that has not even been included on the list of health policy objectives we have been pursuing for the past several decades. What do we Americans ultimately want from our health care system? I'll suggest *healthier people* as the right answer, a choice that isn't even part of the political agenda for health reform. We have spent a rapidly increasing percentage of our gross domestic product on health care in the last half of the twentieth century, but we—as individuals and as a society—are far from healthy.

We probably do have the best doctors and the best hospitals in the world to patch ourselves up when we become ill or injured, but we still end up fairly far down the list when industrial countries are ranked in terms of health indicators. We need to devote more resources to attacking the causes of illness and injury, which likely means devoting fewer resources to traditional doctors, hospitals, drugs, and the like. Which also means that we must make the traditional system as efficient as possible (that is, eliminate waste) so that we will have some resources left over to do things like improve our diets, build safe roads and good cars with better drivers, teach drinkers to be moderate in their consumption of alcohol, get some exercise, get rid of all tobacco products, and the like.

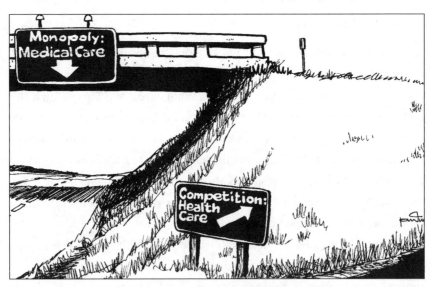

One of the nation's leading health economists, Victor Fuchs, contributed to the evolution of my iconoclastic thinking about health care with his book, *Who Shall Live?*[2] I would like to think that I am taking us one step further with this book, which I might have titled *Who Should Deliver?* However, the most insightful question for the long run may be the one posed by Marc LaLonde in *A New Perspective on the Health of Canadians.*[3] Should our health care system add years to our life, or life to our years?

---

2. Victor R. Fuchs, *Who Shall Live?* (New York: Basic Books, 1974).
3. Marc LaLonde, *A New Perspective on the Health of Canadians,* (Ottawa: Government of Canada, 1974)

I submit that we in the United States are ready to think more about how well we live and less about how long we live. To do so will require completely rethinking the allocation of the resources we are willing to devote to medical care—that is, purposefully reinventing our health care system to do what consumers want it to do. We can begin right now by giving doctors some healthy competition from qualified, independent nonphysician providers.

Index